ESSENTIAL
PILLARS

This Book
Belongs to:

CECISA

So Says
Dr. J.

ESSENTIAL PILLARS

The Three Proven Keys to Success and Happiness

DR. JAY S. GROSSMAN
Foreword by Sharon Stone

Published by Best Seller Publishing®, St. Augustine, FL
Best Seller Publishing® is a registered trademark.
Printed in the United States of America.

ISBN:

For more information, please write:
Best Seller Publishing®
1775 US-1 #1070
St. Augustine, FL 32084
or call 1 (626) 765-9750
Visit us online at: www.BestSellerPublishing.org

To Briar

We have been married for thirty-seven years and counting. There are no words to adequately express my thanks to you for always being by my side and for tolerating those early years when I wrongly focused on one Pillar—money—thus missing out on so much precious time with you. Thank you for teaching me the value of relationships and self-growth.

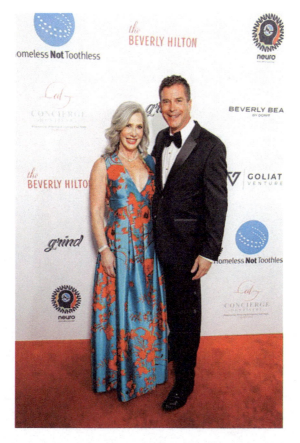

Figure 1: Dr. Briar Flicker-Grossman and Dr. Jay Grossman at the Homeless Not Toothless Gala 2023

Table of Contents

Foreword

by Sharon Stone

When I first met Dr. Jay, I was immediately struck with the thought, "OK, this guy is on the right foot. We can work together and find a path forward." And we have. I have never, ever seen a dentist bring homeless patients to their office. And when I went into Dr. Jay's office and learned he was treating unhoused patients, I was pretty blown away.

So I pitched him an idea about how we could expand his generous humanitarian work with Homeless Not Toothless into an actual working format, grow it ever expansively, and find a path for it that could conceivably help thousands. Well, Dr. Jay has done so much more than anyone ever suspected could occur. He has helped over one hundred thousand displaced humans and changed their lives. He spoke before the California Senate and got the sponsorship of a major TV show and many celebrities.

This does not begin to delve into the enormous individual good things and big things that Dr. Jay has done. So, read this book if you want to feel good, do good, or just do a little bit better with finances, health, philanthropy, or happiness. You will see that it takes a village, and yes, it takes one villager. And that villager just might be you.

https://www.youtube.com/watch?v=pZi02xEXy1Q&list=PL9DD70D903CC98683&index=25

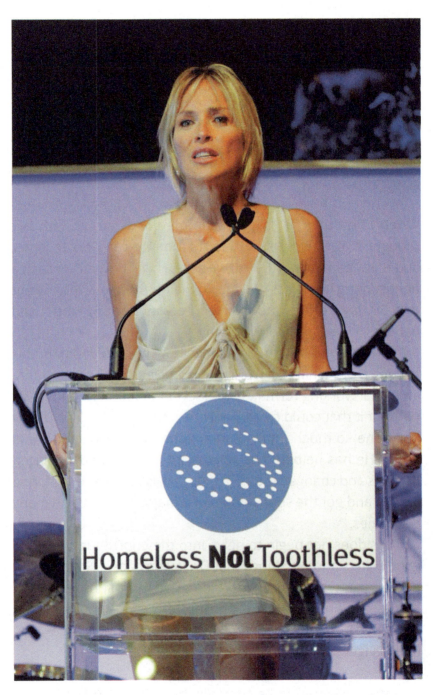

Figure 2: Sharon Stone, Key Note Speaker at Homeless Not Toothless Gala

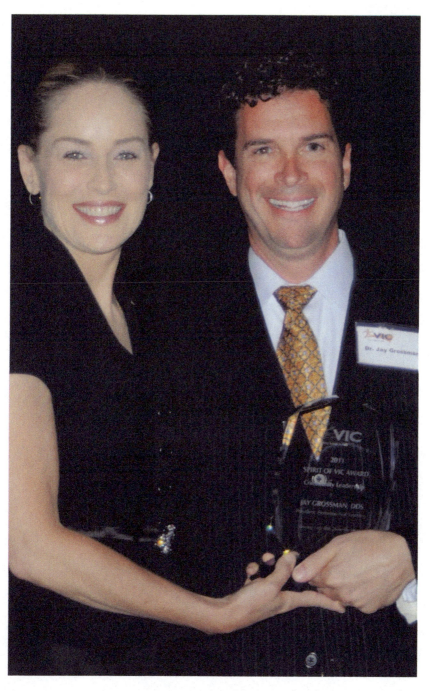

Figure 3: Sharon Stone at VIC Gala, giving Dr J award for work done in starting Homeless Not Toothless

Introduction

Grossman, you'll never amount to anything.

—My high school English teacher, Mrs. Killjoy
(I was too traumatized for too long to recall her actual name.)
Mrs. Killjoy, wherever you are, let's face it: I became a success after all.

Although primarily a concierge[1] dentist by choice and trade, I file more than a dozen tax returns annually for my various entrepreneurial businesses. I've generated nearly $100 million in revenue, I have several patents in health products[2] and exercise equipment, and my brain is constantly whipping up new ideas. Impressive, huh, Mrs. Killjoy? Not quite what you expected back when I was a kid at Plainview John F. Kennedy High School?

Though those are all ways in which I have been successful, they are not *why* I am successful.

I have had the privilege of coaching and mentoring thousands of people, helping them become their better selves. Dozens of others have mentored me, helping to open my eyes to far-flung possibilities in my life.

But that, too, is not why I am successful.

---

1   Concierge Dentistry. (n.d). *Concierge Dentistry*. https://www.conciergedentistry.com/.
2   Grind, (n.d.). *Grind*. https://tinyurl.com/Grind-HNT.

I've been happily married to the same amazing woman for over thirty-seven years. Between the two of us, we have fourteen children. Quite a feat, as you can imagine! But again, that is not why I am the success that my long-ago teacher predicted I would not and could never become.

You see, despite Mrs. Killjoy's dim hopes for my future, I am successful today because I learned—painstakingly and painfully, over the course of many years of research and trial-and-error attempts combined with a hefty dose of humility and self-reflection—that the glory of true success is in cultivating and balancing what I call the **Essential Pillars**.[3]

Sure, I could sit back and count my greenbacks and luxuriate in what I've built for myself, but that would not be authentic or a true self-expression of who I am and the legacy I want to leave. Instead, I want to share what I've learned. That is why I wrote this book. In this publication, I will share with you everything you need to know to begin building the **Essential Pillars** in your own life.

Why do I care? Why would I go to the trouble? Um ... did I mention I have fourteen children? More precisely, I have fourteen kids, eleven grandkids, and all the future children they are likely to usher into the world. If you're a parent, you understand. And if you're not a parent ... you'll understand anyway. I look into fourteen pairs of shining eyes, and I want to leave them a legacy, a meaningful gift—something that may help them and others like them; something I, you, and they can be proud of.

Sure, some parents just write their kids a fat check, but I want my brood to live rich, joyful lives with the know-how to write their own tickets. I want them to have so many inner resources that they will never be without.

---

3 Dr. Jay Grossman. (n.d.). *Dr. Jay Grossman*. http://www.drjaydds.com/.

This book is also an opportunity for me to acknowledge and thank those who mentored me, as well as to share the trials and tribulations that have brought me success—all in the hope that you, the reader, will gain some valuable hacks that may accelerate successes in your own life. From a caring social studies teacher who saw me not living up to my potential to coaches who pushed me to expand and grow, these individuals gave unstintingly of their time and attention to help me, a virtual nobody, realize that I had the right and potential to become a *somebody*.

Wait, scratch that! They already saw me as a somebody, even when I didn't see it myself. I would like to pay that forward and pass along their gift of mentorship to all who read this book and to all who care and dare to live up to their potential.

It wasn't until I turned fifty that everything started to come together for me. That's when I realized I had eight figures in net assets, thanks mainly to the knowledge I had amassed and the "operations manuals" I had put together for all aspects of my life. It was also when I realized I didn't want to keep my secret sauce to myself. I wanted to share it.

Here, I will offer real-life strategies and examples of how to gain mastery in the most critical areas of life. I've included practical tools, suggestions for additional reading if there's an area you want to explore further, and exercises to help you expand on the areas of life that are most important.

In this book, we're going to drill down on money, relationships, personal development, and health, so it may sometimes feel uncomfortable—but I believe such pain is essential. I will divulge personal and intimate thoughts on relationships and money in the hope that you will learn from my experiences and understand that, in the end, we all have "things" in our lives that are uncomfortable and need working out.

Success and happiness in business and personal lives don't happen accidentally. Though some attribute their accomplishments to the mysteries of luck or fate, there's more behind individual achievement than the whims of the universe.

That's why, together, we will dive into each of the **Essential Pillars** and participate in exercises and thought-provoking activities. I believe these activities will give you the desired results in a clear, easy, and concise format. The results will be genuine, repeatable successes.

Consider this book a shortcut to happiness and balance in life. I hope these hacks prove beneficial to you.

Are you ready for the challenge? Let's begin!

The Essential Pillars of Life

Here are what I call the **Essential Pillars** of Life:

1. **P**rosperity
2. **P**eople
3. **P**ersonal

Before we really get into the weeds of how to master, implement, and tend to these **Essential Pillars**, I need to point out that many (if not most) people do *not* experience true success in *all* three Pillars. They may get one right, or sometimes two, but it won't really work if you only address one or two of these three vital areas. Doing so will leave true success just beyond reach.

Plenty of people have a pretty good handle on their health, for example. With occasional blips, they exercise, eat their veggies, watch their weight, and keep the worst of their unhealthy habits at bay. They go to medical checkups, and they get enough sleep—yay, them!

But if they are also in debt or mired in toxic relationships, they are not hitting the mark.

Then there are the fat cats with fat wallets who could buy and sell you and me any day but who are one steak and loaded baked potato away from a coronary incident.

There are countless self-help books out there denoting the exact secrets, rules, or principles for success, joy, time management, wisdom ... you name it; there's a book for it. I've pretty much read them all, so you don't have to. Many offer decent advice, but usually only in one specific area—your love life or your checkbook. Okay, great, but that isn't going to cut it if you're short on time and looking to improve your life in a sweeping, overall way that will put you in good stead now and in the future.

I developed my theory of the **Essential Pillars** with an eye toward *balancing* all three pillars, not just cherry-picking the low-hanging fruit. So, if you only intend to read about and work on *one* of these pillars, you are not likely to achieve the promise of this book. "Success," in my opinion, requires that these pillars are kept in balance, the way financial advisors remind you to keep rebalancing your portfolio as the financial weather changes.

While focusing on only one or two aspects of self-improvement at a time, these books also overwhelmingly recommend finding balance in your life. Balance is the one overarching, consistent theme I have found after spending tens of thousands of hours educating myself through podcasts, books, and classes on growth, development, and money management. They all seem to agree that in life, love, and business, a balance must be found, adjusted as needed, and maintained.

Keeping your life in balance requires active engagement and powering through unforeseen struggles (and struggles are almost *always* unforeseen) while keeping your eyes on the prize—the health and functioning of your life.

BALANCE: THE THREE-LEGGED STOOL

Trained seals can balance inflatable balls on their noses, and daredevils can balance on filaments strung between two skyscrapers. If you want to try any of these activities, you've got the wrong book. That is *not* the kind of balance I'm talking about.

What about the idea of "balance," meaning "equal," like the scales of justice? Having everything tidy, precise, and measured?

Sorry, not that either. When it comes to the messy business of life, nothing is ever totally equal. What is "in balance" for *you* might be way out of whack for your neighbor, and what feels balanced to you on Tuesday may be all wrong for you by the weekend.

Real balance requires setting clear boundaries, so you know when to stop working, start exercising, and start relating to those people who are important to you. It requires scheduling to ensure that the people you love are a priority. It requires leveraging and taking advantage of having a team, and it requires delegating and sharing responsibilities.

No **Essential Pillar** can serve its full function without acting in concert with the other two, and for all three to be in harmony, consider the three-legged stool.

Each leg in a three-legged stool is designed to support your bottom, but it can only do so as long as all three are present. Imagine what would happen if one of those legs is damaged. Maybe it snaps and splinters; maybe your dog is playing fetch with one of the legs, or maybe your kid is using a leg as a sword in a backyard *Game of Thrones*. Whatever the case, when you sit on one or two legs, you fall. Game over!

No one is silly enough to risk the fate of their precious bottom by plopping down on a two-legged stool. So why would you trust your life to only two pillars? Or worse—just one?

Keeping your three pillars in balance means deciding (and occasionally recalibrating as conditions shift) just how much time and energy you need to put into each one. It's a personal, highly subjective weighing of priorities and needs, chosen with care based on your particular circumstances: your relationships, the amount of money you need to support your lifestyle, and your preferred quality of health. I have a black belt in kickboxing and maintain a fitness level to support that, but I am not also aiming to tow a tugboat with my teeth like Jack LaLanne. If I were a fitness guru and not a dentist, I might devote a few more hours each day to strength training and endurance beyond what I do now. Still, wearing breathable synthetic fibers all day isn't important enough to me. I wouldn't be able to run all my businesses or be a good husband and dad if I were forever training for the Norseman Xtreme Triathlon.

Without all three **Essential Pillars** in a kind of balance that works for *you*, the foundation of a truly successful life becomes unstable. This book is intended to ensure that you find your balance. Hopefully, we are seeking to thrive, not just survive.

HOW TO MAKE THIS BOOK WORK FOR YOU

Learn from Failure

"Hey, Dr. Jay," you may be wondering, "what does the road to genuine success look like?"

Glad you asked! The road to genuine success looks like a whole lot of potholes and detours and speed traps.

In other words, the road to success is paved with failure, and I personally have racked up more than my fair share of it. I have definitely hit many potholes while in the process of finding my way—my biggest financial pothole was when I declared bankruptcy in my late twenties. I believe in sharing my mistakes as much as my wins to allow you to sidestep a few of those same roadblocks. Doing so taught me that mistakes, blunders, and downright failures are necessary to get where you're going. They will even get you there faster!

Ironically, I latched onto this wisdom because the first time I realized that most self-help authors were big fans of failure as a teaching moment, I pushed back—hard. I mean, who wants to fail?

It's not that I didn't think the idea had merit—learning from our mistakes makes sense. It's just that I decided, with a big bushel of hubris, that mistakes were fine for *other* people, but *I* would simply do what apparently no one else in the universe had ever thought to do: I would do everything right the first time—done and dusted!

I'm sure you can guess how *that* turned out—mistake after mistake. Blunder after blunder. I trusted the wrong people with my business finances and wound up chasing after a ton of embezzled money. Ouch. But just as those gurus said I would, I learned something from this failure—and the lesson I learned in that case was well worth it. I learned how to screen for the integrity (or lack thereof) people bring to their personal lives before trusting them to have integrity in their business and financial dealings. Although there will always be bad apples, you can toss the rotten ones right away with this simple, no-frills technique. It's like the "waiter rule" for someone you start to date—if they're rude, obnoxious, or patronizing toward the waitstaff in a restaurant, that character flaw is in their DNA and will pop up in other situations.

Check, please!

Where else have failures educated me? Well, how about an example from my personal life? Early in our marriage, I spent too much time on "business" and not enough on family. In fact, my wife wants you to know that this happened so much that

I'm downright lucky she has chosen to forgive me and that our children are still talking to me.

Here's what happened. After working a ninety-plus-hour week (in the 1990s), I returned home hoping to be greeted by a martini and slippers to acknowledge my hard work, only to find a house in shambles. My wife was exhausted after entertaining our three children without a break for her to shower. I was in shock. Where was my cocktail?

I was even more in shock when she turned to me and said, "I don't think this relationship is going to last."

"But why?" I asked, baffled. "I just worked a double shift. I'm making money to build our future."

Briar replied, "That is not all that life is about."

Lesson learned: there are other things in life besides forking up the dough. For a long time, I either didn't believe that or just gave it lip service—but, take it from Briar, money alone does not make for a glowing hearth at home.

Moving right along, did I make any other mistakes? Nothing comes to mind unless you mean the time I bought hook, line, and sinker into a blatant, only-for-fools, get-rich-quick scheme and wound up losing my shirt. From this, I learned what some self-help books do not always make clear: if it looks too good to be true, it is. Also, anything worth having is worth sweating for.

Eventually, through trial and error (but mostly error), I had to admit that many books I'd read were correct on one universal point: failure is an excellent teacher.

Assuming that that is true, here's a question for you: if you could learn from the mistakes of others, would your experience along this road be less painful?

In a word, yes.

That's why, in this book, I will help you skip many avoidable failures by learning from mine. According to Carol S. Dweck, author of *Mindset: The New Psychology of Success*, there is often confusion between *"I failed"* and *"I am a failure."*[4] We need to step outside of that mindset.

Be forewarned, though: you will *still* make at least a few mistakes of your own, but each setback will offer tremendous benefits—as long as you review how and what went wrong, learn valuable lessons from the experience, and put those lessons into action. In this way, failure will help lead you to the ultimate growth you seek.

> *It is hard to fail, but it is worse never to have tried to succeed.*
>
> —Theodore Roosevelt

Get Real

Most people don't have a clear and accurate understanding of what is going on in each of their three pillars. That's because they have not paused to break the pillars down and measure the various components. With the proper metrics, you can analyze whether things are looking up or down.

1. From a financial standpoint, many people don't know their actual numbers, such as what they need to earn each month to pay the bills and how to deal with bills that fluctuate from month to month. Those actual numbers are called your "monthly burn rate" or your "monthly nut."
2. From a well-being standpoint, most people aren't aware of their health stats, such as what's up with their blood

---

4 Dweck, Carol S. (2017). *Mindset: The New Psychology of Success*. Little, Brown Book Group.

work or where their cardiovascular levels fall. There are tons of metrics to look at for your health.

3. From a relationship standpoint, many don't know how their significant other views them or talks about them to their friends. They don't know whether or how much they are loved and valued. This gets a bit trickier: How do you assign a "number" to your relationships? But there are some ways to gauge this.

One reason people often don't know the answers to these questions—aside from being afraid to dig too deep—is because this kind of information usually comes from a third party. This third party may be an employee or customer from a business, a doctor for a health assessment, or a loved one from the relationship standpoint. This involves considering another person's point of view, which can often involve difficult or awkward conversations: "Hey, hon, you'd tell me if I had any flaws, right?" "Are my jokes not funny to others?" "How much do you love me on a scale of one to ten?"

You need to get a set of facts, where applicable, along with a reading of your situation from other points of view to know what standards to set or how to measure or meet them.

Norman Vincent Peale once said, "Shoot for the moon. Even if you miss, you'll land among the stars." The problem is that there are not enough stars to catch you, which is why you need to build, inspect, and quantify your universe.

That which is measured improves. That which is measured and reported improves exponentially.

—Karl Pearson

Think of it this way—you wouldn't buy a stock based on only one data point. You would want to take a look at trends, for example. The more time you have access to this kind of information, the better you can predict the outcome of buying such a stock. That is why it's essential to record your daily progress so you can track the score for each of your pillars over time and see where possible imbalances are at play or threatening to come into play. This requires you to put time aside daily to record goals, track results, and analyze the numbers.

To understand each pillar and how to measure its scale and progress, you need to examine each individually by breaking it down into its components. Throughout this book, you will learn not only the metrics by which you can record your progress but also how to use them to your advantage in your quest for ultimate fulfillment and success.

Make It a Habit

Most people lack habits that result in regular commitment to improvement. Be it exercise, relationships, or finances, many fall short when it comes to doing the work that leads to accomplishment and attainment of a goal. This can easily be mistaken for laziness, but it's merely the lack of an established pattern and system of accountability.

Habits don't form and strengthen overnight. Levels of motivation rise and fall, come and go. The sooner you begin and build on good habits, the smoother and faster your journey will be. Struggling doesn't mean you're not capable, only that you don't have the right tools, knowledge, practice, and systems in place.

In his science-based book *Tiny Habits*, BJ Fogg explains how to pair the smallest of healthy new habits—such as *one* push-up a day—with habits that are already in place, such as brushing your teeth in the morning.[5] It seems simple, but by pairing a painless new habit with an activity that already occurs without much effort or thought, you are piggybacking for a success that can grow at a leisurely rate from one push-up to many, fitting an otherwise intrusive action even into a day with "no time" left for anything. After all, you'll always find a moment to brush your teeth, and it won't hurt you to do a single push-up. Then, when you see how easy and mindless the process can be, it becomes easy to add a second one.

In Fogg's view, a habit becomes easy to create as long as you have the knowledge (you know how to do a push-up), start small (just one push-up to begin with), and can piggyback it onto something you will always do, no matter how pressed for time you are (brushing your teeth).

By the way, Fogg also suggests you reward yourself after doing even that single push-up—not with an ice cream sundae, but perhaps with a mental "Yay, me!" to drop a delicious bit of dopamine into your bloodstream.

If you need more help or encouragement to develop a habit, get a partner in on it for accountability: a gym buddy with whom you have a standing fitness appointment or someone else for a session of "parallel play"—even on Zoom—who is trying to accomplish the same hairy task. Together, you will make it happen.

Take advantage of the modern-day tools and people around you to start and maintain your new habits. I also recommend *The 7 Habits of Highly Effective People*[6] by Stephen R. Covey and *Atomic Habits*[7] by James Clear, along with Fogg's book.

---

5 Fogg, BJ. (2020). *Tiny Habits*. Harvest.
6 Covey, Stephen R. (1989). *The 7 Habits of Highly Effective People*. The Free Press.
7 Clear, James (2018). *Atomic Habits*. Penguin Random House.

Summary for building a habit, according to Fogg:

1. **Commit to it and do it daily for at least thirty days.**
2. **Pair it with a routine habit already in place.**
3. **Say it, write it, read it daily, and share it with an accountability partner.**
4. **Measure it.**

Patience, My Dear

Success takes time. The best way to get rich, fit, or stay in a relationship is in a healthy, sustainable fashion. Yet, there is an endless market for get-rich-quick systems because society has become obsessed with instant gratification, and, ahem, *anyone* can fall into this trap. Didn't I mention I once fell for a get-rich-quick scheme and lost my shirt? Well, at least I looked good shirtless because I'd been keeping up with my health pillar—but that was small consolation.

The same goes for get-thin-quick schemes and the kind of instantaneous "love" promised by so many reality TV dating shows.

Hopping on the latest get-rich/fit/married-quick bandwagon only leads to frustration, and that leads, in many cases, to desperation. If you look up *desperation* in *Merriam-Webster's Collegiate Dictionary*, you will find a photo of me—well, the *old* me. Now, all you'll see is this definition: "a state of hopelessness leading to rashness."[8] As we all know, rashness leads to panic, which leads to making errors. Yes, I said we can learn so much from our failures, but I didn't mean you should start racking them up willy-nilly!

---

8   Merriam-Webster Collegiate Dictionary, (n.d.). *Merriam-Webster Collegiate Dictionary.* Definition of "Desperation. https://www.merriam-webster.com/dictionary/desperation.

There is a time component to everything worth having in life. Take wealth, for example: without a solid understanding of how much time it takes to envision, develop, and grow a business or a financial plan, the expectation of immediate results hijacks your brain—and sometimes your shirt.

Or, think of your health. How many people invest in gym memberships, go once and overdo it, and then limp home, vowing never to hit the gym again? A reasonable fitness program pursued faithfully over time will get you as close to winning the Mr. or Ms. Olympia title as you are likely to come, given focus and genetics. For most of us, that's plenty.

Give the pillars time. Give *yourself* time. Learn to keep your instant gratification monster on a leash for a better life full of unimaginable rewards.

PROSPERITY

1. **Prosperity:** revenue, business, economics, money, financial affairs, income
2. **People:** relationships, communications, rapport, family, significant others, personal friends, and business colleagues
3. **Personal:** well-being, welfare, self-worth, self-help, growth and development, mental and physical health, meditation, exercise, nutrition, time alone, spirituality, purpose and vision, happiness

MY KRYPTONITE: PROSPERITY VS. SUCCESS

Welcome to **Essential Pillar** No. 1—Prosperity. This is my kryptonite, my biggest struggle, in that I have often focused too much on this pillar while neglecting the others.

By most accounts, I am wealthy. But like so many people, I struggle to *feel* financially stable and secure. I am constantly moving the goalposts and have rarely felt complacent about my finances.

Even though I have amassed abundance, I still wrestle with the dread that I need *more*, as if this uncertainty is in my DNA. I recall hearing others say many times that money isn't everything; yet inside, I thoroughly disagreed. What I believed was that money *was* everything.

Growing up, I would often hear my parents arguing over money, a conversation I bet many of you reading this book can also relate to. My father was a purchasing agent for a local electronics company. The job required no travel, was low-stress, and paid a wage that covered the basics. I remember saying to myself, "Why doesn't he work for the larger corporations like my friends' fathers do, to make more money?" I truly believed that the money disputes would end if he'd done that.

As a kid, my takeaway from overhearing their disagreements was that once I became an adult, I would make sure I made "enough" money, and then everyone would be happy. I can see now that it was a wrongheaded, shortsighted view ... but hey, I'm still a work in progress, just like you. We are on this journey together.

Although I have achieved *prosperity*, there have been many times when I did not feel I had succeeded in this pillar. How can that be?

First, let's understand what we're talking about. According to *Merriam-Webster's Collegiate Dictionary*, *prosperity* involves "thriving, especially through economic well-being."[9]

Or, according to the Dr. Jay Dictionary of Everyday Language, we're talking about *money—bucks, moolah,* and *the Benjamins*.

Or is this what prosperity is? Because it turns out that achieving prosperity does not necessarily mean you've got a lock on success.

---

9 Merriam-Webster Collegiate Dictionary, (n.d.). *Merriam-Webster Collegiate Dictionary.* Definition of "Prosperity." https://www.merriam-webster.com/dictionary/prosperity.

Having confessed that this subject is kryptonite for me, I must add that prosperity is truly about more than just dollars. I do have a lot of those, but deep inside—where the child I once was still holds a bit of sway—I'm not always sure I have enough or that I won't somehow suffer from a lack of it in the future. That's why I feel I have to squirrel away the nuts now, just in case.

But while I was squirreling away the nuts, I also had to overcome the nagging feeling that I was raised in what I perceived as poverty and that maybe it showed. I always had the temptation to splurge on show-offy items, like fancy wheels and flashy clothes—anything to "look" wealthy.

Prosperity for some might be a sum in a bank account, but *success* with this pillar, for me, is the feeling that my loved ones and I are safe and provided for. A feeling of financial, psychological, and emotional comfort. Also, it is knowing that when I die, there will be ample funds to pay off any bills and mortgages while leaving plenty of riches for my family to live on.

Some people try to tabulate that into a dollar figure, but how much is too little? How much is enough? There is really no set standard. The "right" number differs widely from business to business and person to person. A mom-and-pop shop will measure financial comfort differently than a multimillion-dollar company on the stock market.

Prosperity isn't about a specific number. It's about the comfort and security money brings to you, your family, and your business. It's about covering the needs and having enough left for the wants. It also certainly involves having money left over for making investments.

In 2022, the average annual salary in the U.S. was around $50,000. At face value, that indicates that if you make equal to or more than $50,000, you're above the norm, and if you make less, you're below it.

However, $45,000 is the average income in Mississippi, and $80,000 is the average in California. Does that mean only people in California experience prosperity purely because they objectively bring in more greenbacks than people in Mississippi? Of course not!

Although $80,000 sounds like a better deal than $45,000, there are other factors at play, such as inflation and the local average cost-of-living expenses. The same sum might stretch a whole lot further in Mississippi, where you can buy an extra car or a bigger house with a smaller mortgage than someone making twice as much living in LA. *Now,* who's livin' large?

What I'm saying is that prosperity—as well as the attributes of the other two **Essential Pillars**—can exist independently of success.

PROSPERITY EXERCISE 1:
What Do You Want, and Why?

What is *your* definition of success? Often, people assume success means having more money than God or becoming so famous you can't go to a restaurant without diners rising to give you a standing ovation.

The *Merriam-Webster* dictionary has a different idea. It says *success* is "the favorable or desired outcome."[10] This means that if you set a goal, *whatever it is,* and achieve it—voilà! You are a success.

Perhaps you are a new business owner and think you would die happy if just *one* customer were to purchase your product or service on opening day. In this case,

---

10 Merriam-Webster Dictionary, (n.d.). *Merriam-Webster Dictionary.* Definition of "Success. https://www.merriam-webster.com/dictionary/success.

once you survive your "successful" opening day, life goes on. You will need to come up with a bigger vision of success.

The real issue with your Prosperity pillar is to decide not just on a dollar figure but also on a desire or aim you have for your work, or business, or for whatever way you plan to spin off a profit. Then, you can make a step-by-step plan for how you can go about attaining it.

I strongly suggest you get at least one coach for each pillar, especially the pillars in which you are weak.

Write down the answers to these questions: [11]

1. Why do you want coaching?
2. What do you want to get out of it ?
3. What is *your* story about money (there is never enough, my parents were spenders, I live paycheck to paycheck)?
4. What would it mean to you if you had financial integrity (defined as more coming in than going out while living a lifestyle that you choose)?
5. What is your definition of success?
6. Can you follow a routine of consistently looking at your finances and recording the results?

You always want to go back to the reason "why." Why do you want more money? Why do you want authentic relationships? Why do you want to be in better shape? The "why" will be your strongest motivator for getting the result.

---

11 Dr. Jay Grossman. (n.d.). *Prosperity Exercise 1, Success defined.* www.drjaydds.com.

Your "Nut" in a Nutshell

Now that you've come up with your vision of what "success" would be like for you in this pillar, you can look at the numbers that might support that vision. Is there enough? Is there too little? What is your actual situation?

If you recall our discussion about "getting real" and using metrics to measure your progress, it's time to apply that knowledge as you assess your Prosperity pillar.

Even if you have an accountant, or a whole raft of them, it is still important for you to have an awareness of your personal and business finances. Mistakes happen, and when they do—and they will—you never want to take the chance of something going horribly amiss. Your finances seep into every aspect of your world; a single weak link in the chain can make the fence collapse, and the longer mistakes go unnoticed, the more they compound and the more difficult they become to fix.

A reminder: the nut (or burn rate) is the baseline sum you need in your account for bills you simply cannot avoid or lower. This goes for your personal nut as well as your business's nut (if you own a business). My philosophy, shared by many, is that you should not pay off more debt or invest in anything new until you have a minimum of three times (3x) your burn rate in cash savings. There's another reason why financial awareness is so important: you can't know what 3x your monthly nut is without understanding your monthly nut in total.

The Bare Minimum

Why is "3x" the magic number? That's the formula many use—myself included—for ensuring there's no stress in managing living expenses during periods when there is *no* income, such as during the COVID-19 pandemic, when many businesses had to close for months. Having a safety net brings tremendous comfort, as it allows you access to funds if your business slows, you find yourself between gigs, or you become temporarily unable to work.

Without knowing how much 3x your monthly nut is, it would be hard to ensure you have the proper backup fund for emergencies. When people ask me, "Dr. Jay, what's in your to-go bag in case of emergencies?" I tell them: "Three times my monthly nut!"

Okay, I do not literally keep wads of bills in my to-go bag. And, in the interest of full disclosure, no one has ever asked me this question. Still, I would like to think that if they *did* ask, this would be my answer because that would be a good lead-in to a conversation on the value of having financial awareness.

Unless you have stored up savings equivalent to at least 3x your monthly nut, you cannot reasonably explore investment options for even more financial growth. First things first. And this 3x goes for your personal life and every business you own as well.

In a business, customers are your primary source of profit, but they aren't the only source. You need a solid financial foundation and security net before you can branch out and invest in other areas.

Leave nothing out when evaluating your finances, and ask an accountant or trusted advisor questions about the flow of money. Sometimes, problem areas are more easily spotted by a third party—especially one who doesn't stare, scowling, at the same spreadsheets every day.

Remember, *self-preservation* leads to poverty, while *self-investment* and *smart business decisions* lead to wealth.

In your financial life, do you know your monthly nut offhand? In both personal and business finances, that would be how much money goes out to pay for absolute, immutable essentials. Betting on the ponies doesn't count—no matter what you think, that is not considered an essential.

Are you covering that nut each month? To find out, you need to know *exactly* how much money is coming in.

If the two figures are close—money in, money out—that is the break-even point, and there is nothing left over to play with or invest. I call the amount you need to breakeven the Minimal Acceptable, or "MA." This is the least you need to get by each month.

Knowing your MA means being in touch with reality—and, as the movie title suggests, *Reality Bites*. Knowing the truth about your situation is crucial and sometimes painful, but it can also be a relief. The pain of acknowledging your real-world situation can galvanize you into taking positive action to improve it. After all, the purpose of pain is to get our attention so we can fix things before they get worse.

Is pain getting your attention right now in certain areas of your life? Or has living with low-level pain become the unhappy status quo for you? I am not encouraging you to try to eke out a living on your MA. That's not fun. You want—and deserve—more than that in life.

That's why I advise being careful not to fall into the trap of aiming too low and living in pain on the bare edge of "minimal." You want to aim higher. Personally, I like playing games that challenge me and force me to grow and expand, which means I rarely hit all of my goals. And when I *do* happen to hit all of them, it's usually a sign that I'm playing too small. This is a habit that I had to get trained on—it's called "failing forward." It means that I play games where there is a good chance I will "fail," and I then learn from those mistakes. I learned what was missing, which, if present, would have had me hitting the goal, and then I played again for that new goal with the tools I learned from the failed experiment.

The only way to know what's what in this pillar is to understand your MA threshold and make realistic plans to surpass it, along with a contingency plan in case things go haywire.

Then, and only then, can you play the game of financial abundance.

Gross vs. Net

Before you embark on Prosperity Exercise 2, here's a little recap of two terms you need to understand: gross revenue and net income.

Gross revenue is the money your business receives for goods or services before taxes and other deductions are calculated. If you are getting a salary check, it is the top number before taxes are taken out.

Net income is what you take home after deductions and after taxes.

Objectively, both are important statistics, and gross revenue is vital to your financial awareness on a business level—but on a personal level, the number you want to focus on is your net.

Gross revenue feeds your ego. Net revenue feeds your family.

PROSPERITY EXERCISE 2:
"What's So"

You're probably reading this book because you do not want to settle into the rut of being "just okay." Good for you! With that in mind, I invite you to participate in what I call the "What's So" exercise: getting a true, accurate accounting of your finances.

In a moment, I will have you gather some information—and please don't skip this step, or you'll be cheating yourself! Statistics are essential because they are the only way to determine your MA and thus have a foundation for setting future goals.

Success in this pillar requires you to have an entirely transparent view of the following:

- How much money is coming in (and from where)?
- How much is going out (and to whom)?

Don't scratch your head and say, "Oh, I know the answer; it's approximately ...". No "approximately" allowed—find and write down the actual numbers. This information needs to be clear, reproducible, and reportable—meaning that if you were sitting down with me for a coaching session, you could show it to me.

You know what's even better? Record this information in Microsoft Excel or on similar spreadsheet software.[12] Some of you out there who have successfully avoided working with spreadsheets all your life are groaning, but

---

12   Dr. Jay Grossman. (n.d.). *Prosperity Exercise 2, the "What's So."* www.drjaydds.com.

trust me, it's worth it. In my experience, those who run from spreadsheets really run like the dickens—which will serve them well when we discuss maintaining cardiovascular health in the Personal pillar. The hard truth is that an aversion to Excel and similar apps may be holding you back from some of the success you seek.

If you are one of those people who have never used a spreadsheet, consider the benefits of learning: it allows you to adjust numbers easily and create what-if scenarios without having to do more arithmetic. Most spreadsheet software allows access to the file on your phone, so you'll never be without it when you need to make changes on the fly. The internet offers a wealth of resources to help you learn and become more proficient, not to mention the endless instructional videos you can find on YouTube. I'm not asking you to do pivot tables or power queries—basically, just learn how to enter and add up a column of numbers.

If you're not ready to use a spreadsheet program, do this exercise anyway! Write it down on a napkin if that's all you have handy. Don't use any excuses—you don't need to devote two years to earn a certificate in accounting before you can count your money.

Let's start with the amount of cash coming in. This should be relatively easy if you're employed full-time and are either working consistent hours at a set wage or are salaried. It becomes a bit more challenging if you work for yourself and your income varies. If that's the case, record the average and keep it conservative: instead of working off that one windfall month, average out the totals of the past six months.

On the expense side, as discussed, you need to know your monthly nut—meaning every necessary, recurring expense. That includes rent, mortgage, insurance, car payments, alimony, loans, food, travel, gas, and minimum payments on all debts. Leave nothing out!

Fixed costs for running most businesses also include payroll, rent, insurance, accounting, and legal costs. These are "fixed" because you must pay them no matter what, and they tend to remain about the same, month to month. They likely bear no correlation to your sales figures (they have to be paid every month regardless of sales), and you need to know them in order to run any business.

The nut for your personal life also involves fixed expenses, but you will want to supplement your overall financial picture by seeing where else you drop your dough. For example, although obviously you have to eat, food is not technically a "fixed" expense since you can tighten your belt at some times and splash out on fancy restaurants at others. Keep items such as food, clothing, entertainment, repairs, doctor visits, dry cleaning, home supplies, and so on, as a separate list you can compile by averaging out what you spent in those areas over the past year.

Here is an example from one of my businesses: a few lines that clearly articulate the vendor, the date money is due, the way it gets paid (by check, automatically charged to a credit card, or automatically withdrawn from the bank account via ACH—which stands for Automated Clearing House, a network that processes electronic bank-to-bank money transfers), and the amount due. This information helps me quickly look at the upcoming week and immediately see the expected number of withdrawals.

Vendor	date due	type of payment	amt due
Dental Intelligence	20	autopay	$ (299.00)
Kaiser Health Insur	21	autopay	$ (403.86)
"Spectrum" Time Warner tele/internet	22	autopay	$ (132.00)
911 Porsche	24	ACH	$ (1,971.38)
Viva Marketing	25	autopay	$ (2,790.00)
Fidelity Pension	25	autopay	$ (3,822.00)
A Slice of PR	25	autopay	$ (500.00)
SBA EIDL loan	26	ACH	$ (2,509.00)

If you have not yet compiled your financial records for this exercise—perhaps because you were hoping you could just read through this section and avoid *doing* it—it's time to roll up your sleeves and get busy. Go find those records and take however much time you need to calculate your "What's So."[13]

1. What is your total net income (the amount you receive after deducting taxes)? Check your previous year's tax returns to see how much you typically pay in taxes. If you bring in multiple income streams (also known as horizontal income), record each with the name of the company or entity on its own line. (A single source of income is called vertical income.)
2. What are your expenses? List all your expenses, one per line, just as I did in the example above.

Now comes the fun part! What can you cut out, what can you cut back on, and where can you find resources

---

13 Dr. Jay Grossman. (n.d.). *Prosperity Exercise 2, the "What's So."* www.drjaydds.com.

to put into savings for your 3x? What additional income can you bring in? Can you increase revenue from your current job? Can you take on something part-time to bring in extra money until you hit your 3x?

This exercise is best done in tandem with your significant other or with a financial/business coach.

Money Outflow

Now that you know "what's what," you might wonder, "But where does all that money go?" Money seems to have a nasty habit of slipping through one's fingers.

There are four categories through which money can flow *away* from you: Burn Rate, Taxes, Debt, and Investments. Knowing there are four buckets helps me tremendously when I study my cash flow. Burn rate can consistently be decreased by tightening the belt on expenses. Taxes can be reduced by discussing tax-saving strategies with the right accountant or tax advisor. Debt is a killer, so if you ever want financial freedom—a life without chains—you really must eliminate it. I will share some debt-tackling strategies in more detail later.

Finally, my favorite area into which money can flow is investments. Remember, a job is where you work for money, while investments are where your money works for *more* money!

Burn Rate

How fast your money disappears. This is the money you "burn through" each month—so if you're popping champagne corks all day long, you're probably the kind of person who burns through money rapidly. But it doesn't take a lot of Lamborghini Gold

Extra Dry Prosecco to see your cash ebb away too quickly for comfort as you pay expected bills and juggle unexpected ones.

You have a certain amount of control over how much money flows through this category. You can start by reducing your overall spending and expenses where you can. Fewer trips to Starbucks, perhaps—or at least order the "tall" and not the "venti" size. Or more home cooking and less takeout food—not to mention paring back on more significant items such as cars, rent, and travel.

To calculate your personal burn rate, you need a living, breathing, updatable record of your monthly nut—which you already did in Prosperity Exercise 2 (the "What's So" exercise).

Over the next month or so—hey, it's a journey!—take a hard look at your budget. How much do you genuinely *need* to spend each month to live? Carefully and honestly determine which expenses are necessary (e.g., the roof over your head) and which can be chucked or at least lowered. And remember, this exercise in cutting back is not necessarily something you will be doing forever; it's designed to free up money *now* for your 3x savings.

Taxes

Taxes are what you pay to the government in return for various services that keep society's wheels turning. Paying taxes is a necessary, legally binding, annual process that needs to be tracked and planned monthly.

I know you hate paying taxes. Everyone hates paying taxes. Still, a lot of good comes from it—and I'm reminded of that every time I see an emergency services vehicle in action. Yes, it's frustrating when the government wastes funds, and it's irritating that the more you make, the more you owe—as if you're being punished for your success. Nevertheless, we all must pay taxes. To help you with that, there are two million words in the tax code that explain it.

Oh, wait, that does not help anyone at all! Not a single person I know—at least, who is not a certified public accountant (CPA)—can even pretend to understand all the twists and turns in the IRS tax code, and it's not worth anyone's while to go through all two million words to try to make sense of them.

The good news is that only a few dozen pages in all that verbiage speak specifically to tax incentives or breaks that may benefit you. These are legal deductions that incentivize people to make certain investments the government wants people to consider.

That is why choosing the right accountant is so important. It would be best if you had an exceptionally competent team to decipher all those rules and regulations. Having solid tax-saving strategies with your accountant's advice is crucial. Learning about tax breaks is the kind of knowledge that literally pays off.

For example, there are benefits to limiting your W2 income if you own your own business and are taking money out as a draw instead. When you own a business, there are legitimate write-offs that are not taxed; that's one of the reasons I am a big fan of owning a business. There are similar benefits to renting your home to your business for up to fourteen days a year—you can get a tax break for that rental. (The "Augusta Exemption" is the popular name for Internal Revenue Code Section 280A(g).) There are health savings accounts (HSA) that allow you to put money for health care expenses into a fund you can access in retirement, and there are insurance vehicles that offer tremendous tax savings as well.

I'm not the tax expert here, but I know which experts to call, and they are just as good. Seek professional advice and build a list of influential people you can rely on to ensure your taxes are accounted for.

Debt

Debt refers to what you owe in incremental payments over time. Debt is a necessary evil for most people when they start off in life, but only up to a point. Then it's just plain evil!

Too many people stay in debt for life. Some debts, such as a home, a real estate investment, medical bills, education bills, or a business loan, can be considered reasonable. These debts are on assets that gain value if treated well, which will help boost your credit rating and net worth.

On the other hand, many debts aren't fiscally sound—such as a boat you hardly ever take out on the water or that credit card whose carrying charge is so heavy it can be used as an anchor on that boat you hardly ever take out.

Imagine, for a moment, what it would be like to be free of debt, to have no money allocated to chipping away at an amount you owe. It took me decades to realize how satisfying and fulfilling this would be. When I finally paid off all my real estate investment debt and "owned" my rental properties, I reallocated my newly freed-up money that was no longer going toward that sinkhole called "paying the bank" toward new investments, a new home, and travel. Being debt-free allows you to take money tied up and dangling just beyond reach and earmark it for other vital areas. I currently have debt on my home and a car, and I am paying this off at an accelerated rate with cash flow from my passive assets.

If you currently have debt—and most people do—you'll have monthly expenses in this category. You can eliminate the category by paying off all your debts. Easier said than done, right?

Many conflicting theories exist about whether carrying debt is good, bad, or acceptable. I believe it is permissible to carry limited debt on items that bring you a return, such as a business, education, or real estate. That means paying off your mortgage, as there is no return on your home financially while you carry that onerous debt. Assuming your home appreciates over time, there is no return on your home simply for living in it—no return on investment (ROI)—which is why, for me, carrying a mortgage is something I avoid if at all possible. Once you have your 3x in the bank, my advice is to start saving for passive investments, which are the stock market or real estate, and then take the profits from these investments to pay off the home debt.

You'll have a monthly expense in this category if you carry debt. But I strongly advise against taking on *new* debt until and unless you have at least 3x your burn rate in savings.

PROSPERITY EXERCISE 3:
Pay Off Debt

How much money is disappearing because of your debts?

On your Microsoft Excel spreadsheet or similar spreadsheet software, list each debt by the debtor's name, plus the amount due, interest rate, and minimum payment due.

Next, sort the file by interest rate so the debt with the highest interest rate is on the first line. Sorting columns in spreadsheet software is quite simple and easy to learn, so hey, none of that whining!

If you must, keep paying the minimal amount due on all the debts each billing period, but also put any extra money toward paying off the *highest* interest-rate debt until that loan is retired, especially if the rate is above 4.5 percent. Loans under this amount might be okay to keep if you've filled the bucket of investments that yield 5 percent or greater.

For example, here are my loans, sorted by interest rate, with the highest interest rate on top:

Loan Name	Interest rate	Balance	Monthly payment
Chase Mortgage	4.63%	$ 731,873.00	$ 5,036.00
Porsche 911	3.09%	$ 65,344.00	$ 1,971.00
Bank of America Loan	2.65%	$ 119,543.00	$ 4,011.00

Here are my options:

Option One: Pay down the Chase mortgage at an accelerated rate, as the interest rate is higher than that on the car and bank loans. Any extra funds in any given month, after I pay off my monthly loan, will go toward paying off the highest-rate loan. But, as you can see, paying off that balance will take many years.

Option Two: Pay off the loan with the lowest balance. Using the same example above, if I paid off the Porsche car payment, I could use an additional $1,971 per month toward paying off the highest-interest loan.

Both theories hold water. It comes down to how many months or years it would take to pay off the lowest-balance loan and whether choosing Option Two versus Option One makes more sense. Use the *Essential Pillars* Debt Spreadsheet[14] to help you see what your debts look like.

---

14   Dr. Jay Grossman. (n.d.). *Prosperity Exercise 3: Debt Spreadsheet.* www.drjaydds.com.

INVESTMENTS

"Investments" refers to the commitment of resources intended to achieve more significant benefits in the future. Once you cover your burn rate and put aside 3x that sum to cover emergencies, pour any extra money into investments that can grow into more income, businesses, Lamborghini Gold Extra Dry Prosecco (if you must), and more everything.

Robert T. Kiyosaki, in his famous book *Rich Dad Poor Dad*, says there are four ways to earn money:[15]

Employee	Big Business
Small Business	Investor

He intentionally presents it in this format, as the left-hand side offers little, if any, leverage. The right-hand side is where true financial freedom enters the picture. Let's take a minute to look at the tax rates between the left- and right-hand sides of Kiyosaki's diagram.

Employees pay between 10 and 37 percent of federal tax and 1 and 12 percent for state tax, so it is possible to pay 50 percent of your tax earnings (if you make over $500 thousand in W2 income). You heard that right; *half* of your income goes back into taxes as an employee at high-income levels.

Small businesses typically pay 30–40 percent in taxes after write-offs, and you pay the full 15 percent for self-employment tax.

Big business pays a flat tax of 21 percent on profits! You need to have over $7 million in revenue or over $10 million in assets and have over 500 employees to qualify as big business.

---

15 Kiyosaki, Robert T. (2022). *Rich Dad Poor Dad*. Plata Publishing.

But look at the tax break—30–50 percent on the left-hand side of the diagram (employee and small business) to 21 percent tax for big business!

Finally, there is the investor, who pays between 0 and 15 percent by using tax-advantaged accounts, insurance products, retirement accounts, borrowing against their own assets, and utilizing long-term capital gains, which is only 15 percent, as compared to ordinary income, which is up to 37 percent!

I find this simple diagram brilliant. When I first saw it, I was on the left-hand side, an employee. I was a dentist in the Navy, making around $30,000 a year with no extra cash in my pocket and no ability to invest. Plus, I was working for somebody else (the U.S. government). My first realization was that I could start a small business and eventually become an investor, as I wanted to avoid being involved in big business at that time.

As a small business with little money to invest, I got involved in multi-level marketing (MLM). This industry type requires you to enroll friends and family in buying products or services from you directly, cutting out the brick-and-mortar stores and basically giving you the profit from the savings of not having a storefront.

MLM schemes can be dicey. After all their hard work, people have gotten snared in pyramid schemes or made little money. I advise you to enter something like this with great care and only after doing due diligence. I'm not saying that the route I took to wealth is exactly the route you should or need to take.

Fortunately, the several MLM companies my wife and I got involved with were solid and ethical and offered fantastic products. After a few years, we had saved enough to buy our first home. Then, we saved enough to invest in our first rental property.

Kiyosaki's diagram stuck with me. I realized I needed to move to the right-hand side of the chart and gain more leverage.

I would need to become an investor.

The Four Investment Buckets (Asset Classes)

Whenever I think about expanding my financial reach, I ask myself: Which of the Four Investment Buckets do I want to be in, which bucket do I know well, and which bucket do I need to get educated in? Let's look at the four buckets in detail (business, real estate, securities, and insurance products).

1. Business
The first place to consider is your career or business. You can't bring in revenue to use toward other investments without having a source for that revenue, and a business can be a great source.

Once your business is stable and consistent, generally within the first few years, you can explore other investment buckets. Before you diversify, build the first business with the proper tools to run by itself. Otherwise, that business is more likely to fail or produce marginal results.

2. Real Estate (RE)
Renting out or flipping properties after first sprucing them up can be a great investment option. Another RE alternative is looking at the building your business runs out of. Suppose there's an option (and you have the financial capability) to purchase the building through which you already operate a business. In that case, you won't have to worry about the prior owner selling it from under your feet. Also, when you want to retire (or if you ever want to sell the business), you will still have

an income from the property, which you can rent to the new business owner.

You can hop into the next bucket once your real estate consistently brings in money.

3. Securities (Stocks and Bonds)

There are so many stock options, but to start with, you should look at index funds, which are painless and the easiest way to get going until you have enough money to consider allowing a broker to manage your portfolio. Once you have amassed $50,000, find a reputable stockbroker with a successful investment history; that way, you will have a more substantial likelihood of a positive return, and you won't have to spend an enormous amount of time learning how to make your own wise trades and checking stock tickers. I heavily invest in an S&P index fund with no fees and have a broker to deal with my other investments. One of my favorite index funds is the Vanguard S&P (VOO). This stock can cost about $500 or so a share (in 2024), so it is available to nearly everyone. Perhaps it will take months for you to save up for a share, or maybe you can buy several shares per paycheck—either way, this is a great way to start having your money make money.

4. Insurance Products

As with stocks, it's best to seek out a professional who knows insurance inside and out and can confidently invest your money in the right kind of portfolio. The goal with insurance investment—with all investments—is to guarantee "permanent profitability," with stable passive income coming your way even into retirement. Igor is the point person in this bucket. Igor is quite a character; you'll learn more about him later!

What Goes Where?

You've got your cash. You've got your four buckets. What to do with it?

Some recommend pouring everything you can into a single bucket. Some have experienced tremendous success with this method, but it involves the risk that makes my breathing get ragged. Most people, including me, subscribe to the idea of diversification, of investing a little into each of the buckets.

Vertical income is revenue from a single source, whereas horizontal income is revenue from many sources. Ultimately, I believe that multiple streams of income are necessary to be diversified and fiscally safe.

When lecturing, I often show side-by-side photos of Virgin Galactic entrepreneur Richard Branson and Berkshire Hathaway CEO Warren Buffett. Both are successful billionaires, but they follow opposite investment philosophies.

Branson owns more than two hundred companies, whereas Buffett believes in being like a postage stamp—sticking with one thing from the moment it's affixed to the envelope until the moment it's delivered. Neither method is inherently right or wrong. It's a matter of how much and what risk you will tolerate.

Investing always involves some degree of risk. If you put all your eggs in one basket, you might win big, but it's possible they will all break—meaning no more omelets for you.

I'm somewhat risk averse and prefer the Branson theory of multiple businesses. I like to invest a bit in each of the four buckets, then rinse and repeat. After one business, property, brokerage, and insurance product, I start back at the top and look for another business, property, brokerage, and insurance product.

What is *your* risk tolerance? Do you want to diversify or put all your eggs into one big basket?

Pay Yourself Before Diversifying

This simple concept of Four Investment Buckets makes planning and diversification easier, leading to permanent profitability, in which finances no longer make you pull your hair out.

Many first-time business owners funnel all their incoming money back into the business. They believe it's the only way to get out of the red and gain financial longevity. In the process, however, they often forget to account for their personal financial needs.

This is another reason why understanding the monthly nut is essential—not just for a business but also on a personal, at-home level. You don't want to risk losing your house to keep your business afloat.

Here's the rule: Pay Yourself First. No need to question it. Just accept it.

At first glance, it may sound strange, even greedy. Trust me, there's a reason behind this wisdom. How does that work, though? How do you pay yourself first, ensure your business has all its needs taken care of, *and* ensure you've covered your monthly burn rate?

In his book *Profit First*, author Mike Michalowicz recommends that at least 10 percent of your income be immediately set aside for long-term savings. That money will be reinvested into the four buckets, and you will pay *yourself* before anything else.[16]

This is where the plan of diversification comes in—but note that diversification does not mean splitting that 10 percent into

---

16   Michalowicz, Mike (2013). *Profit First*. Penguin Random House.

four portions of 2.5 percent apiece and putting it into each of the four buckets simultaneously. Instead, it means starting with one investment in one of the four buckets, then rotating to the next investment, the next, and the next. Once the cycle is complete, start from the beginning again, just as I do: build a business, buy real estate, invest in stocks, and buy insurance products. Rinse and repeat.

Here's more of what Michalowicz has to say about how to carve out that 10 percent for yourself and what to do with it.

If you own a business, open five bank accounts and name them as such:

1. All Income/Holding (100 percent of all income)
2. Profit/Invest (10 percent or more)
3. Fixed Expenses (30 percent)
4. Variable Expenses (30 percent)
5. Owner/Operator Expenses (30 percent)

All income must flow into the All Income/Holding account. *Immediately* transfer 10 percent or more of that income into the Profit/Invest account.

Then, transfer 30 percent into the other three sub-accounts, following the 30-30-30-10 rule. The "30" refers to the *maximum* percentage of expenses for each category. If your expenses are more than 30 percent in each category, you either pay people too much or do not generate enough business top-line income.

The 30-30-30-10 rule for business expenses:

- Up to 30 percent of the total income goes toward fixed expenses, like staff payroll, fringe benefits (e.g., insurance benefits), taxes, and rent.

- Up to 30 percent of the total income goes toward non-payroll expenses, known as variable expenses, including supplies and advertising.
- Up to 30 percent of the total income goes toward your salary or the person you delegate to run the business.
- Ten percent or more of the total income goes toward profit and long-term investments.

The 30-30-30-10 rule makes it easy for you or your accountant to determine your gross income. You must look at all the money that floods into the holding account.

If you get a paycheck, the formula changes a bit. Begin with the "10" of the 30-30-30-10 rule. Take at least 10 percent of each paycheck and move it to a savings account for long-term investments. This is crucial, as you need to develop the muscle to manage 90 percent or less of your income to pay all the bills.

If you do *not* own a business, open four bank accounts and name them like so:

1. All Income/Holding (this is the account into which your paycheck auto-deposits)
2. Ten Percent Profit/Invest
3. Burn Rate
4. Debt Repayment

Next, twice a month, move money into the accounts based on the schedule you have set up.

At least 10 percent goes directly into the Ten Percent Profit/Invest account: immediately transfer 10 percent from All Income/Holding to this account on payday.

That leaves 90 percent of your pay toward your Burn Rate and Debt Repayment. This is why budgeting and knowing your monthly burn rate is crucial.

For example, let's say you have a salary of $4,000 or $2,000 auto-deposited twice a month. Immediately put $200 (10 percent of $2,000) into the Ten Percent Profit/Invest account. That leaves $1,800 every two weeks, or $3,600 monthly, dividing the Burn Rate and Debt Repayment accounts.

Notice that there is no "tax" account if your income is only from being an employee. As an employee, taxes are already taken out from your paycheck. Your goal is to eliminate the Debt Repayment account and decrease your actual Burn Rate so that, eventually, you can put more than 10 percent into the Profit/Invest account. This is the *only* way to get financial freedom—to have money to invest in passive income.

I am always amazed when I coach salaried workers who receive significant raises and still seem to find a way to spend it all! How is it that even when extra money comes in, one sees more ways to spend more?

Note: your sub-accounts are not piggy banks—do not borrow from them! Suppose there isn't enough money in the All Income/Holding account to pay yourself first. In that case, your business has a big problem—either you're not generating enough income, your expenses are too high, or your eyes are bigger than your wallet.

It's essential to identify this issue immediately and, if necessary, haul in a professional for a consultation to help you fix it. If you don't bring in enough money to cover the bills, you must decrease your expenses and increase your revenue. It's pretty simple—work harder or longer, get more customers for more inflow, or tinker with your costs to lessen outflow.

Remember that personal and business expenses fall into two main categories: fixed and variable.

A business's **fixed costs** include rent, salaries, insurance, property taxes, and utilities. These expenses occur regardless of whether the business is open for business or on vacation.

Variable costs include commissions, supplies, food, cost of goods sold (COGS), and postage. These costs vary monthly based on your and your customers' needs.

In dentistry, the ideal goal is to have fixed costs at under 30 percent of the pie and variable costs at under 20 percent, leaving 50 percent for profit. This would be a well-run dental practice with a 50 percent total overhead. The national average in dentistry is a 70 percent overhead *before* the owner/operator (the dentist) account is paid. So, the 30 percent remaining in dentistry is the dentist's salary, which is why most dentists who own a practice have really just bought themselves a job.

What's the industry standard in your field? Comparing your profit to the industry standard will tell you whether you run an efficient business.

The 30-30-30-10 rule is for getting started running a minimally effective business. Once you get a handle on that, you can move to a different rule: the 30-20-50 rule. This is the ideal ratio for a well-run business:

- Thirty percent of total income goes toward fixed expenses.
- Twenty percent of total income goes toward variable costs.
- Fifty percent of total income goes toward profit and long-term investments (now you jump from 10 percent going toward investment to 50 percent).

Here's a summary of the subtle differences between account names in business vs. personal:

Business Accounts	Personal Accounts
All Income/Holding	All Income/Holding
Profit/Invest (10% or more)	Profit/Invest (10% or more)
Fixed Expense (30%)	Burn Rate (incl. Fixed and Variable)
Variable Expense (30%)	
Owner/Operator Expenses (30%)	Debt Repayment

In business, the "burn rate" is broken down into fixed and variable expenses, whereas in personal, it is all lumped together and called the burn rate. One could argue that the total of fixed and variable expenses in a business is the business's "burn rate."

ELEMENTS OF BUSINESS SUCCESS

Now that you understand where your money's going, the wisdom of paying yourself first, and how to pay off your debts so you can begin investing, things may become more evident. But wait! How is your business faring? Is it strong enough to get you where you can start investing in the Four Investment Buckets?

Most workers in the U.S. are salaried employees whose paychecks depend on their job description, company culture, and their bosses' whims. This leads many workers to want to branch out on their own.

That's what I did—many times over. While I encourage others to try it, I still have to point out that starting or investing in a business is not for everyone.

For example, just because you love deli sandwiches doesn't mean you should open a deli. In *The E-Myth*, Michael E. Gerber begins with the example of a baker who is excellent at baking apple pies but doesn't know how to operate a cash register;[17] the lesson is that you shouldn't start a business solely because you enjoy making the product. A lot goes into running a business; if you don't have the right people and systems, baking a prize-winning pie will be the least of your worries.

Loving something is excellent, but you need a lot of puzzle pieces in place before starting a business.

Are you still interested? Great!

In that case, keep in mind that there are only three fundamental areas for any business:

1. Sales and marketing, which provide the business with clients.
2. Operations are how you run your business—standard operating procedures (SOPs). It would be best to have a book available to your employees that tells them everything from turning on to turning off the lights and everything in between.
3. Finances and administration manage infrastructure, staff, and money flow.

---

17   Gerber, Michael E. (1998). *The E-Myth*. Harper Business.

Mentorship, Coaching, Partnership

Now, let's break down the overarching categories of the elements of business success.

Four out of five businesses fail in their first five years due to a lack of planning, mentorship, cash, and accurate reporting of monthly expenses, as well as a lack of a complete understanding of statistics and how to run a business—and those are just a few of the possible missteps.

When you look at that list, I'll bet you nod your head at some of the items: you need enough start-up cash. Right, it's crucial to have a plan.

And then you come to "lack of mentorship," and you screech to a stop, like a needle flying off the record on the turntable. You're probably thinking, "Who needs mentorship? I'm smart enough to get by on my own!"

Can you hear me making the sound of the game-show buzzer, indicating you got the answer wrong?

Think of sports. Have you heard of anyone making it to the Olympics without a coach? Most professional sports teams have multiple coaches. No athlete would think, "Hey, I'll just bat a few tennis balls around and then trot myself over to Wimbledon."

Why is coaching so well-known and accepted in the field of sports but much less so when it comes to the pillars of prosperity (business), people (relationships), and personal (well-being)?

Being both a mentor and a mentee is invaluable. As a mentor, you give to someone who wants to learn while, in turn, cementing your comprehension of your teachings. First, observe, then do, then teach.

As a mentee, you receive training, motivation, advice, support, and help in setting goals, driving toward them, and ultimately attaining success. Getting intelligent, third-party input is always helpful. Learning where your blind spots are and how to avoid mistakes is critical. Mentors in all three **Essential Pillars** keep you grounded, humble, and teachable. I have multiple mentors in each pillar, as I want to grow, expand, learn, and become bigger than I know myself to be.

These days, I'm eager to bring more people into my life and businesses. I would much rather have a robust and reliable team and leverage myself with people who are assets. Learning to be a team leader takes training—who you *hire* is not always as important as who you *don't fire*. Leaders should work with people who deserve to be led and deserve to grow. You can lead a horse to water, but you can't make him balance your books!

Going into business with someone you love (perhaps a family member or friend) is appealing for many reasons—but if you want or need a business partner, it's best to choose with your head, not your heart. A good partner needs the necessary skill set for the job (preferably one that complements your own instead of merely duplicating) and the personality required for handling inevitable trials that will pop up along the way. With eight billion people on the planet, you have more choices than just those sitting around your dinner table, so take your time and choose the right partner. Hey, that goes for the People pillar as well—marry the *right* person!

Business management, let alone ownership, isn't for everyone. If you're new to the business, what support structures do you have in place to manage the areas with which you are unfamiliar?

I once formed a partnership with a family friend. It ended in a lawsuit. I couldn't believe that someone I liked, someone whose kids' weddings and bar mitzvahs I'd been to, would steal from me. My wife had had doubts about him years before I took him on as a partner, so it was graceful of her not to say, "I told you so," once it all came crumbling down. My estimate of this individual is that he was a 2 out of 10 in all three pillars, which was a red flag that I had clearly missed. He was unsuccessful in business and his marriage, which was toxic to our partnership as he lacked integrity. I chose to overlook it for far too long.

Fortunately, the court awarded me a big fat check, which I used to pay off my car loans. After that, I remembered the pain and sweat I had put into building that company every time I took my Porsche out for a spin. The pain I went through when having to pursue a lawsuit, coupled with the years of time investment, was onerous and a waste. Be careful and thoughtful about who you partner with.

On the other hand, my friend Zak—a personal trainer, actor, and stuntman—came to me with several business investment ideas, including funding a movie, renting raw land for filming, and obtaining a patent on exercise equipment. This is someone who proved himself to be reliable and trustworthy over time, so I was happy to contribute and show my support. Although none of those businesses brought in Elon Musk-style profits, it was an easy, happy, and ultimately profitable partnership. We sold nearly one million dollars in exercise equipment—the movie and the raw land have not yet produced results. However, it is so pleasurable to work with Zak that I don't mind if all the businesses we attempt are not home runs; the experience is excellent, and there are no regrets.

You can partner with a friend or loved one as long as you do your due diligence.

Don't Compare

Comparison is the thief of joy.
—Theodore Roosevelt

Are you better than this one? Not as good as that one? Taller, shorter, richer, poorer? Who cares? Your job is to show up and hit it out of the park, make a difference, do your best, and stay focused on your mission and vision. The *only* person you should compare yourself to is the "you" of yesterday.

I'm not as good a basketball player as Michael Jordan; then again, I am several inches shorter, and anyway, I'm a dentist. It's okay to strive toward *your* personal best, as long as it's your personal best and not someone else's.

Don't you want to be a better iteration of yourself? That is why the best person to compare yourself to is the person you were yesterday.

Clear Mission, Vision, and Core Values

How can you achieve success without a solid picture of what you want to achieve and how you *want* to be perceived by others, including co-workers, employees, vendors, friends, and clients? The answer is to have a clear Mission, Vision, and Core Values.

A **Mission Statement** describes the overall objectives that you are committed to achieving. What is the comprehensive summary of your company's purpose? How do things stand now? Are you fulfilling your purpose today?

A **Vision Statement** is a declaration that clarifies where you see your business going and what you hope to achieve in the long term. Where do you want to go?

Finally, **Core Values** are the personal ethics that guide you in decision-making. They frequently are the same for your business and your personal life.

Goals, meanwhile, are the specific actions you take that will, more likely than not, lead to you *achieving* your Mission and Vision while upholding your Core Values. That is why you need to have it all written down. Goals are the dreams, the finish line, and the result you are playing for.

Your actions reveal who you are. Look at your schedule, and you can see if you are committed to creating your life or if you are at the mercy of headwinds and circumstances. It takes time to become successful, and how you plan and use your hours today determines your success tomorrow.

You need a clear and concise Mission Statement that everyone who works with and for you knows by heart. It must contain a Vision of where the company is going and build upon a solid set of Core Values. You must maintain a stellar reputation and show off those opinions online so the world knows who you are. Testimonials give others an instant snapshot of how well your **Mission, Vision, and Core Values (MVCV)** are being executed. Especially in our modern age of business, people care about what's going on behind the scenes.

For example, here is my MVCV for my dental practice and those of some other companies as well:

1. My dental Mission: empowering, protecting, and inspiring your smile.
   - Ben and Jerry's: making fantastic ice cream.
   - Google: organizing the world's information.
2. My dental Vision: continuity of care, one-stop shopping for all your dental needs.
   - Ben and Jerry's: making the world a better place.

- Google: providing access to the world's information in one click.

3. My dental Core Values: integrity and professionalism.
   - Ben and Jerry's: advancing human rights.
   - Google: focusing on the user; all else will follow.

My MVCV is posted in my office and is a screensaver on my computers. Staff and patients can see it all the time.

If you are running a business, I strongly suggest you make your MVCV concise and visible and ensure you and your crew can see it daily to align with its message.

CORE VALUES DICTATE VISION

To formulate your business Vision, you need to define your Core Values.

An example of Core Values would come from putting together a wish list of your ideal employee. Your Core Values statement would include exemplary service, commitment to the client, excellent attendance, and loyalty.

What will your holiday speech to your staff look like? Even if you are at the beginning stages of building a business, consider writing it out and using this speech as a vision board guiding you toward your Core Values.

Consider the Core Values in this excerpt from my holiday party speech in 2018, after thirty years in business:

Over the past three decades, we have generated tens of millions of dollars of business. We've accumulated some of our industry's best technology and treated more than 15,000 patients. But enough with numbers; let's talk about our people. Our top priorities are commitment to one's job, integrity, and treating patients with the best technology, care, and compassion. We are open to new ideas and new policies that will better us as providers and provide better results for our patients—these things are what define us and make us extraordinary and different. This is our special sauce.

Other examples of Core Values are honesty, openness to coaching and constructive feedback, continuous self-improvement, being unafraid to speak out when faced with a problem, attention to detail, teamwork, enthusiasm, tenacity, and so on.

Another way to examine your Core Values is to contemplate: What is your business's higher purpose (aside from making money)? What niche does it fill?

Here are some further questions to help define your Vision:

1. What are your Core Values—those profoundly ingrained principles that guide your actions?
2. What is your core focus, which you are passionate about, and what is your reason for being?
3. What is your ten-year target in terms of financial or client-attraction goals? Goals are like magnets—they attract what you really want, so make sure your goals are something you really want.
4. What is your marketing strategy—how does your business allocate and channel its promotional efforts?
5. What is your one-year game? "Game technology" equates business to a sport. In basketball, for example, games have a time limit, and in business, it is crucial to have the same. Your one-year game, then, might be something like: "By the last day of next year, I will have fifty new

clients, one million dollars coming in, and 40 percent profitability," and so on.

6. What is your three-year game?
7. What are your quarterly goals?
8. What are the issues or challenges that are stopping you from winning your game?

McDonald's SOP: The Gold Standard

In 2020, McDonald's hoovered up over $19 billion in sales. How did they accomplish that when you know you can make a better burger in your kitchen, their seats are murder on your bottom after ten minutes, and the servers who take your order do not look old enough for the big-kid rides?

The company's continued success is largely due to its famous standard operating procedures (SOPs) manual, which breaks down every step of running a McDonald's, making everything run like clockwork, down to the frying of the last french fry. The manual clearly produces results, despite what you may think of the quality of the food!

The McDonald's SOP manual is the gold standard of SOP manuals. It is to McDonald's what the Gideon Bible is to hotel rooms—always within reach and always reliable. McDonald's replicates the manual and sends it to its 37,000 stores worldwide.

The reason I know so much about the McDonald's SOP "bible" is because I worked at one of the eatery's franchises when I was in high school. The SOP manual was pretty impressive. It detailed every step of the daily routine, and it was how I learned how franchises and other successful businesses operate: find the right formula, then duplicate it.

Let's see if I remember my training: the top of the bun is called the crown, the bottom is the heel, and for the multilayered

Big Mac, the middle piece of the bun is called the club. There's a condiment gun to squeeze out dollops of the "special sauce." There's a technique for properly folding the sandwich wrapper.

It was my very first job, flipping burgers. Without that SOP book to guide me until it became second nature, I would have been toast.

Wait, what am I saying? I *was* toast! I got fired. Not a great introduction to the business world, but it wasn't my fault.

No, really! It wasn't!

Do you know how badly they pay kids at these fast-food places? At least at Mickey D's, we got to eat for free—at first—until I tested the limits of that particular perk and ruined it for everybody.

The deal was that if you worked longer than four hours, you earned a meal break. According to the SOP book, you were ostensibly allowed to help yourself to anything in the warming bin that was ten minutes old or older. After ten minutes, they threw it away.

Remember, I was a growing boy. Teenagers have to fuel their growth spurts. I'd go on my break, have six Big Macs, four large fries, and a few fish sandwiches, and wash it all down with three shakes.

The new owner was not pleased to see my overflowing tray.

"Grossman, get over here," he barked. "What do you think you're doing?"

"I'm working an eight-hour shift, so I get a break," I explained. "And everything I took was at least eleven minutes old. Ancient."

You could see his eyes ticking over my items as he tallied them in his brain.

"That's fifteen dollars' worth of food there," he observed.

Remember, fifteen dollars back in the Dark Ages of my teenage years was a big sum. I thought maybe he was impressed. I mean, my appetite was impressive.

The next day, there was a sign over the clock-in machine: New Policy—$3 Food Limit.

"Excuse me," I said, approaching the new owner. "What do we do if we're going on break and there's more than three dollars' worth of old food that's otherwise getting thrown out while your employees are hungry? Do we just waste all that food?"

"Clock out," ordered the new owner.

"But I just clocked in!"

"You're fired."

I'm not too proud to admit I walked home crying after that—not only had I been fired from my first job, but I was also still hungry!

I soon realized I could turn this incident around to my benefit. I vowed right there and then that I would never work for others and that I would treat my future staff with dignity and respect. In a way, I owe it to that jerk that I became an entrepreneur.

I think I kept my promise because today, I have staff members who have been with me for thirty years. And they, too, have easy access to our SOP manual, just like at McDonald's, except without the burgers. It includes step-by-step instructions for everything, from turning the lights on first thing to shutting down at the end of the day. A properly realized SOP serves as a training manual for new hires and recent promotions, and it should also be available for reference at any time to ensure consistent, smooth, hour-by-hour operations. It's a living document, meaning that it changes and grows and gets amended as often as needed. I back up the current version annually, so I have a historical document of my SOP over the past thirty-plus years.

Consider this: If you buy, in 2024, an established franchise that dates back to, say, 1955 (when the first McDonald's opened), and you are following a really well-constructed SOP manual, is your opening day really just Day One of the business? Or are you reaping the fruits of a business that has been going great for nearly seventy years?

Despite everyone's familiarity with McDonald's and how they have prospered, many businesses are in danger of failing because they do not have (or forget to consult) a detailed SOP manual.

Hint: If you don't have one, the easiest solution I can offer to building one is to have each employee document their everyday tasks over a week. This will become the "job description" for that position, an important component of the SOP. Put time aside to work *on* the business, not just *in* the business. Schedule time to fill in the missing parts of the SOP, starting from turning on the lights at the beginning of the day to switching them off at the end. Also, once they document their "job description," have them sign it for purposes of ownership. This way, if they are not doing their job, you can remind them of what they authored—and if there is still no improvement in their performance, you have a basis for letting them go.

Loyalty and Customer Experience Tracking

Customers can make or break a reputation, which ultimately can cut off your revenue. That's why you want to create and maintain a built-in loyalty base of customers who love your products or services and who love *you*.

Why must they love *you*? Isn't it enough that they hire you or purchase the hand-stitched tea cozies you're selling on Etsy? Isn't it enough that your business offers reliable, caring customer service and that the Better Business Bureau has not come after you with torches like the villagers trying to get Frankenstein's monster to leave town?

Sorry, no. It's not enough that they love your tea cozies. They also need to have a sense of who you are—and *like* you for it.

The method I follow is philanthropy—it ensures that my customers know of my commitment to larger causes than just money and my desire to make a difference in the world. Let people know who you are and what you care about. Doing so helps create super-loyal customers, and they are the ones most likely to provide positive reviews and testimonials that spread the word.

And, as with everything else in your business, track it! You need a method of tracking customer opinion to learn what you're doing right and what still needs work. You can't please everyone, but if customer feedback flags something in particular consistently, you don't want to miss it. I respond to all online reviews, good and bad, and I try never to make people feel as though they're wrong.

Responding promptly and positively will demonstrate that this is a business that cares.

Commitment to Improvement

Businesses that never strive to do and be better do not get far.

That doesn't mean that all long-lived businesses are perfect—far from it. But longevity depends—at least, in part—on some kind of plan and will to improve. In my dental practice, I review our mission every day before I see my first patient to ensure that I remember what I'm promising and make sure I deliver.

Consider the adage: "The customer is always right." Is that your mission? Your vision? Weren't we all taught it's true that customers are always right?

My problem with the "customer is always right" thinking is that it doesn't include a commitment to change. It's more like an attitude of: okay, whatever.

Also, customers are *not* always right, and you cannot earn client respect by giving in to their every whim. You don't learn how better to tend to their needs by slapping a bandage over the issue. If there's a disagreement, I suggest acknowledging it before choosing whether you still want to work with that person. If not, ending the relationship in a clear-headed, professional way is essential.

For example, I had a patient who was always thirty to forty-five minutes late for dental visits and insisted on being seen. Even so, I allowed it twice. When I realized that this is who this person was—consistently late, which affects my ability to see other patients on time—I terminated the relationship after discussing the concerns with the patient and seeing that they were not willing to commit to being on time. I went back to my core values—integrity and professionalism—and clarified that I do not have integrity with my other patients who show up on time if I continue to allow this one patient to throw off my schedule. Remember my definition of integrity: doing what you say you will do in the time frame within which you say you will do it.

The way I ended this business relationship was by saying, "I am so sorry that we are not able to meet your needs, as our schedule does not allow for it. I am happy to refer you to three quality dentists in the area who may better suit your schedule."

For those who have an issue with finances, for example, I might say, "It seems that we are at an impasse. We have very different ways of looking at the value of this situation, and I'm sorry we cannot seem to find common ground. Would you prefer to talk about it and see if we can come up with a solution, or would you like assistance in finding another office that may better suit your needs?"

A statement like this may be appropriate to use with a customer who you simply cannot please, no matter how many plates you spin in the air. It might also help with one who disrespects you or your staff. I have only had to trot out this technique a few times over the past three decades, and the relief and support of my staff for letting inappropriate clients find another dental office went a long way. My core values of integrity and professionalism—coupled with some of the finest quality dentistry in an environment that is friendly, courteous, and respectful and that runs on time—have allowed me to practice dentistry in a manner that is becoming more of a unicorn in my field. By that, I mean I don't take dental insurance, I charge a respectable fee for my services, and I provide an experience that has patients return and refer. I am finding this type of environment more challenging to locate elsewhere within the medical community, where waiting for a doctor for hours has become the norm, and the amount of time a doctor spends with a patient is shriveling.

This is one of the reasons I started a referral network of physicians who cater to more of a concierge-style of medicine—which, again, supports my ever-growing practice: Doctors Who Care.[18]

Your overall plan and philosophy must include the intention and execution of future improvement. Otherwise, it's nothing but a good idea scribbled on a scrap of paper.

---

18   Doctors Who Care. (n.d.). *Doctors Who Care.* https://thedoctorswhocare.com/.

Campaign Tracking

You always want to track the return on investment (ROI) of campaigns. In other words, you want to track how often an ad runs and how often the phone rings because of that particular ad. How many appointments or sales did that ad generate? Is there at least a 3x ROI, thanks to that ad?

Here is an example of how I track my ad spends:

income total from ads	$7,749.00	$9,937.00	$22,032.00	$38,770.00
cost that month	$5,013.00	$ 6,681.00	$ 5,635.00	$12,452.00
ROI	155%	149%	391%	311%
	24-Jan	24-Feb	24-Mar	24-Apr

Since I am looking for at least a 3x ROI, a 3x ROI, the ROI needs to be over 300 percent. So, looking at this, you can see that the ads in January and February fell short, so I dropped those platforms and focused on the ones producing results.

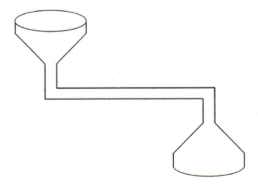

This image—aside from being an artistic masterpiece you will surely want to frame and hang on your wall—is my conception of a marketing funnel. I use this simple diagram in my life daily, be it for business, back when I was dating, or in *any* area where I want to produce results.

To keep a business humming along, you need an active marketing campaign that brings in new business and keeps the funnel filled at all times: new leads and opportunities come into the wide mouth of the funnel. You manage, massage, and nurse them. The final result, the sale, comes tumbling out the other end.

Or, let's say you want to get married. You need enough people coming into the funnel to date. You need to go out with them enough times to learn who they are, what they like, and whether the two of you are compatible. The final result comes out the other end of the funnel—your soulmate!

People are forever complaining about not having enough money. Again, I draw this simple diagram and ask the following questions:

1. What are you doing to bring in leads, get customers, and ensure these are the right customers for your business?
2. What is the level of service you're providing to them? How often are you "touching" them with appropriate emails, letters, and in-person meetings? What is their experience of you during this time?

Drop all your efforts into the hopper, and out the other end of the funnel comes the right kind of customer: one who pays your fee, stays loyal, and refers others to you.

This is not rocket science. It's math. Quality in = quality out.

Now, let's say you're pouring tons of leads into the funnel, and nothing's coming out. What gives?

In this case, you may need to look at the quality of the service or product you're offering. Do your tea cozies fit your customers' teapots? Also, look at the quality and message of the advertising or marketing tools you're using to attract customers. It can be hard to thread that needle because the services or products on offer and what the clients want vary from business to business and person to person. Not all ads and promotions work across the board. Sometimes, even the same business in different locations needs to tweak an ad that worked great in the first setting.

If I can save you a few bucks here, let me offer this: do not throw money into campaigns blindly! The point of any promotion is to make back what you paid in for the advertisements—and more. I like to set my sights on bringing in at least 3x the ROI.

Only by tracking your campaigns will you learn the formula for what draws the right kind and number of clients to you. I hope by now you see that if you want to improve at something, tracking everything is important—be it revenue, expenses, advertising campaigns, calories in/out, or number of dates with your significant other.

Clearly Understood Finances

Just by reading the first part of this book, you have probably come a long way. But for those of you who are still not feeling entirely financially savvy, you have two options: either get educated and comfortable with your finances or partner with someone who *loves* numbers and can boil it all down for you. If you want to be in business, you *must* have knowledge of the financial documents I am about to detail.

Make a Statement

As you learned earlier by doing Prosperity Exercise 2, the "What's So" question—knowing how much money is coming in and going out—is the first step. But there is much more behind understanding your business's finances; indeed, there are all kinds of statements you'll need to read as part of knowing where and toward what your money is going.

The basic reports needed for any business are P&L, balance sheets, and cash flow statements. We're going to break that down to the very basics, but again, I strongly encourage you to refer to books or online tutorials on basic accounting principles so that you will not feel lost at sea.

Profit and loss (P&L): also called an income statement, this document may look complex, but it's basically Revenue – Expenses = Profit or Loss. If there's more coming in than going out, you have a profit. The opposite, of course, is the situation you would like to avoid.

Examine your P&L on a bimonthly, quarterly, *and* yearly basis, tracking the data over days, weeks, months, and years. A P&L statement looks complex until you start to know what you're looking at, which only comes with repetition. This is a habit you must trot out at least bimonthly; otherwise, you have no control over understanding the past to improve the future. Only by knowing the current status of my business on a moment-by-moment basis can I make the right adjustments to get back on track.

In Prosperity Exercise 2, we discussed fixed costs. On top of those, you still have other costs involved in driving sales. Those additions are known as variable costs and include advertising, sales commissions, and utilities. These vary month to month, depending on how much you put into areas such as advertising. And as sales go up, commissions go up, too.

It's vital to compare periods of time for which a P&L is ideal. Comparing quarter to quarter or year to year will show what's happening to your business. Is it becoming more or less profitable? Are your costs increasing? Look for the "story" embedded in the numbers.

Before we look closer, let's get some vocabulary straight:

Assets include your cash in the bank, accounts receivable, the value of your supplies and inventory, and long-term investments and real estate. Your assets are what you own in total.

Liabilities are what you owe, including accounts payable, salaries, taxes, and loans.

Technically, there are two types of liabilities. If the business owes to a lender, it is called a liability; if the business owes to the owner, it is called equity.

Equity includes stock in the company, as well as retained earnings—which are profits you haven't yet taken out of the company.

Now, let's take a look at your P&L statement. Are you looking? Hey, why are you turning pale?

I'll bet it's because you see several lines that are each labeled "profit." Here, let me explain.

There are three kinds of profit: gross, operating, and net.

Gross profit is simply your total income minus the cost of goods sold. (Costs of goods sold are also called COGS; simply subtract your direct fixed costs.)

Operating profit is your gross profit minus your overhead expenses (subtract your direct and indirect costs). This is also known as "earnings before interest, taxes, and amortization (EBITA)." This number is very important because the value of a business you want to sell is based on a multiple of the EBITA. Overhead—all the costs of running your business—is perhaps the most important tool to understand because if you can control the amount of money that's going out, it becomes much less important how much money is coming in. Think about this: a business grossing $3 million at 90 percent overhead makes $300,000, whereas a business grossing $1 million at 50 percent overhead makes $1.5 million. (The gross number feeds your ego. The net number feeds your family.)

Net profit is what people traditionally think of as "profit." Also known as the "bottom line," it has additional items subtracted, including interest and tax expenses. This is profit, free and clear, to put into your wallet.

A balance sheet is a snapshot in time of all that you own (assets), all that you owe (liabilities), and all your equity (assets minus liabilities). This is for a fixed moment in time—a specific date—as the numbers are always fluctuating. In short, this is a snapshot of your net worth. Consider having a balance sheet not just for your finances but for all three pillars in your life so you always know your current status.

The challenge with a balance sheet for nonmonetary pillars becomes a bit trickier. For example, if you are in a committed relationship and want to put a number on the quality of that relationship, how would you do it? You may want to consider asking your partner what grade *they* would give you and start tracking that number!

A balance sheet gives you a picture of the health of a business at any given time. At the bottom, you will see the totals of your assets, liabilities, and equity. It's called a balance sheet because they must be in balance; the assets must be equal to and balanced with total liabilities and equity.

Again: Assets = Liabilities + Equity (and they must balance out)

A cash flow statement is a summary of how money is coming into and out of the business. Accountants make this a bit difficult by having two types of accounting methods: cash or accrual. Here, I'll be discussing only the cash method, which is simply about recording money the moment it's received and the moment it's paid out. This statement shows the trends over a period of time.

The beauty of the cash flow statement is that it's identical to your P&L (income statement) when you use the cash method. With the accrual method, there is an additional statement that does *not* match your P&L. Most businesses are better off opting for the cash method of accounting.

I recommend QuickBooks for tracking your money. It runs all these reports for you or your accountant. Using the online version is best, as the company frequently updates the software. With this cloud-based method that you can access from anywhere, you can keep your finger on the pulse of your business.

Data and Metrics: You Can Count on It!

Without data, you have no idea where you are, where you're going, or if you're on track. That's why measuring results through a scorecard, also called a dashboard, is crucial. Measurable activities—key performance indicators (KPIs)—provide a simple and concise way to get an overview of all your company's data.

Numbers are everything. When you assign numbers to every single job position, it cuts out the murkiness of determining whether the job is being done right.

For example, the people who answer the phone could have a number to measure their effectiveness. For example, picking up the phone within two rings or less results in a good score, while every ring past the third one, or every missed call, brings their score down. Further, what percentage of those calls result in a sale or in a client making an appointment?

The same goes for elsewhere in business. If you can measure it, you can move it. Assign a number to everything that moves you toward your ultimate goal. It gives you something to manage and manipulate.

Financial Acuity

One of my favorite podcasters, Reese Harper of *Dentist Advisors*, came up with a fourteen-point system[19] for measuring financial acuity. Although he designed it for dentists, these measurements cross over to other fields. These fourteen items are crucial for understanding the Big Picture of your finances, and I recommend keeping such a list handy and updating it regularly:

1. Cash savings (should be at least 3x your monthly nut).
2. Real estate holdings (this is a category where you can have "good" debt, meaning a mortgage, as long as the rent exceeds expenses—then you are cash flowing. I'm a big fan of this type of debt).
3. Value of your "stuff": cars, jewelry, and so on.
4. 401(k) retirement fund.
5. IRA retirement fund.
6. Personal spending (super important to know because money can so easily seep away without your noticing it).
7. Insurance (disability, personal article floater for jewelry, life, homeowners, long-term care, auto, earthquake, renters, workman's compensation, medical, cyber, etc.).
8. Profitability (what's left over after expenses and other outflows are subtracted).
9. Investments.
10. Business value (what you could sell your business for).
11. Liquidity (how much cash is in your pocket if you sold everything today).
12. Taxes.
13. Net worth (assets minus debt).
14. Debt management (how you are set up to pay off your debts).

---

19 Dentist Advisors. (n.d.). *Dentist Advisors*. https://dentistadvisors.com/.

LEADERSHIP

If you run a business, you are ultimately accountable for everything that takes place within it, including the occasional employee who messes up. Leadership requires you to have excellent PR skills because if you can't train them for the position you need, you must set them free to find employment elsewhere—and this can be painful.

Jocko Willink and Leif Babin, in their book, *Extreme Ownership*, talk about how everything is your responsibility when you take on leadership.[20] Blaming others makes you look weak and takes away from your ultimate responsibility, which is to ensure everyone on your team is properly trained.

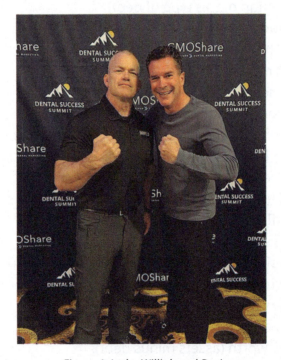

Figure 4: Jocko Willink and Dr. J

---

20   Willink, Jocko and Leif Babin, (2015). *Extreme Ownership*. St. Martin's Press.

If a person who works with or for you makes a mistake, the first question you may want to ask yourself is: "Where did I fail to train them, or why did I not fire them if they're not trainable?" Or, if they were assigned to an incompatible, business-style expectation, it's up to you either to change their job or change them out for someone better suited for the position.

If you want to influence people in a way that generates a consistent, positive result in business and in life, you must step into the shoes of the inspirational leader you know you can be—someone who can motivate, take charge, and delegate.

Three Styles of Business: All In or Spread Out

When it comes to operating a business, there are three primary styles of running a business. If you are not strong in all three, then you need to either learn the others or get partners or a board of advisors who are strong in the other styles.

1. **The Historian:** someone who looks to the past and collates statistics. Data collection and analysis are important—as well as learning from the past—but this style struggles to have a vision beyond the events of yesteryear and set active goals that work for today and in times to come. This style focuses on how or why something did or did not happen and on patterns and trends.

2. **The Technician:** someone who thrives on tinkering with and solving today's problems. This style is excellent for day-to-day management and systems, as its focus is on the here and now and on what needs immediate attention to keep daily processes flowing.

3. **The Entrepreneur:** someone who lives in the future—not on dreams and gas fumes but through written goals and

plans for achieving them. This style focuses on what's next and relies on the Historians for data points they can repurpose into new strategies for Technicians to use today and for everyone to use tomorrow. This style, in my opinion, is the one to consider if you want to lead others in a highly successful business. As we mentioned before, you need to work *on* your business, building and tweaking it, as much as you work *in* your business.

These three styles have different strengths and weaknesses, all of which are vital parts of business operations. It's important to know which style you wear well and to recognize the pros and cons that come with the territory. Historians and Technicians may not be prime business-owner material, but they are still necessary parts of the business-style trinity.

Failing Forward

Failing and failure are two entirely different concepts.

Most people see "failing" as an inherently bad thing. However, *failing* at something is only as bad as you make it. Failing means "a usually slight or insignificant defect in character, conduct, or ability," per Merriam-Webster.[21] The key words here are "slight" and "insignificant," meaning that "failing" naturally lacks intensity. Thomas Edison failed over 1,000 times at inventing the light bulb!

The problem lies not in *failing* at something once, or twice, or even three or more times, but rather when your failings lead you to throw in the towel completely and reach the point of utter *failure*.

---

21 Merriam-Webster Dictionary, (n.d.). *Merriam-Webster Dictionary.* Definition of "Failing." https://www.merriam-webster.com/dictionary/failing.

This is not to say that giving up should never happen. Sometimes, it's wiser to cut your losses and not throw good money after bad. It can be as necessary to eventual success to shut certain things down (businesses and relationships) when they're dead as a doornail as it is to learn from those failings. Failures should be followed by thoughtful tweaks, pivots, and improvements.

Successful people actually fail more often than unsuccessful people! And most of them will gladly tell you about the many times they experienced failings that helped them get to where they are today because they didn't allow those *failings* to transform into *failures*.

Both success and failure leave clues. It's up to you, always, to evaluate both. This is what's called *failing forward:* learning from your mistakes and making improvements. That's where you experience the breakthroughs. As long as you embrace each instance of *failing* as an opportunity to learn and grow and try again, you'll never become a *failure*, especially if you have strong goals and habits backing up each step along your path to success.

You want intensity? Try failure! From Merriam-Webster again: the "omission of occurrence or performance."[22] It's an utter absence of follow-through, according to the Dr. Jay Dictionary of Random but Crucial Thoughts from Dr. Jay's Brain, which has yet to find a publisher (don't know why not, especially when I have such a great book title that just rolls off the tongue).

Consider looking at failures in the same light as going to the gym to strengthen a muscle. The more stress you put on the muscle, the more pain you get, and the more the muscle rises to the challenge and strengthens.

---

22   Merriam-Webster Dictionary, (n.d.). *Merriam-Webster Dictionary.* Definition of "Failure." https://www.merriam-webster.com/dictionary/failure

For me, I want to fail gracefully, meaning I have safeguards that are not catastrophic in nature. A safety net, if you will—a Plan B. For example, I have four patents, and none of them to date have been wildly profitable. I did not throw my last dollar into them, nor did I neglect other responsibilities while working on them. If they fail, I will either abandon them, sell them, or reinvent them while, at the same time, continuing to support the businesses that are successful.

PROSPERITY EXERCISE 4:
Failing Forward

Here's an advanced-level assignment. Think this through: how can I fail *bigger* than ever before?

Go ahead, consider it. Start from the position of: "I cannot wait to see how I'm going to fail at this task, what I will learn from it, and how I will come out the other side happier and more successful!"

Remember, it's better to be a failure at something you love than to be successful at something you hate.[23]

Essential Pillars Prosperity Exercise 4, Failing Forward

What games are you playing that are crucial to your expansion?
What games are you playing small at?
What games if you were to play really big, and perhaps fail at hitting the goal,
        would still expand you and get you closer to your goal?

Crucial: Goals must be specific and measurable, with a planned date of achievement, i.e.,

        I want to cut my expenses by 50% for the next 6 months
        I want to increase my income by working overtime by at least 20% more by next month
        I want to have at least one date night per week with my significant other immediately
        I want to have 3x my monthly nut in savings by Christmas
        I want to have all my finances on my "What's So" spreadsheet by this Sunday
        I want to start a savings account for my child's education by next quarter
        I want to limit my credit card spending to $1000/m starting today
        I want to be debt-free by next summer

23   Dr. Jay Grossman, (n.d.). *Prosperity Exercise 4, Failing Forward.* www.drjaydds.com

Consider this exercise if you are struggling financially: Play a game to cut your expenses by 50 percent next month, a feat that seems impossible when you are living paycheck to paycheck. What if the results are that you can reduce your expenses by 25 percent? That means you failed at your goal of reducing expenses by 50 percent, but you were able to cut down by 25 percent. There is a win embedded in that lesson: you failed forward.

Working Genius

The right person in the right seat at the right time is essential. People have their own special and unique talents, which are often applicable to very specific roles in the office. Each person needs to understand their job description, be excited about it, and have the capacity to excel at it.

In addition, there needs to be a system of accountability. Who does what? How do we know it got done? Or done well?

Each job position ideally comes with four to six daily accountability items. This ensures that team members are managing their part of the mission of the business. In my practice, every team member has a list of their obligations for the day. They check them off and run them by their supervisor.

The 6 Types of Working Genius: A Better Way to Understand Your Gifts, Your Frustrations, and Your Team, by Patrick Lencioni, contains a brilliant parable about how successful businesses and relationships use people's innate talents and stay clear of areas that most frustrate them.[24] If you have expertise in a

---

24 Lencioni, Patrick (2016). *The 6 Types of Working Genius.* BenBella Books, Inc.

certain area, the author calls this your genius. If you're decent in an area, he calls it competence.

And if you don't thrive at all in a given area, he calls it frustration.

Lencioni defines six areas of work: wonder, invention, discernment, galvanizing, enablement, and tenacity. These, along with knowing your staff's forte and assigning tasks within their specialty, help produce extraordinary results while reducing burnout.

1. The genius of **wonder**: the ability to speculate and ask the right questions.
2. The genius of **invention**: generating ideas that seem to come out of thin air.
3. The genius of **discernment**: instinct, gut feeling, the ability to assess an idea even in the absence of data.
4. The genius of **galvanizing**: rallying and motivating people, building teams, and inspiring people and enrolling them to take action.
5. The genius of **enablement**: providing support and assistance; being naturally inclined to help others achieve their goals; team-building.
6. The genius of **tenacity**: the ability to push things across the finish line. People in this category get things done right and see tasks through.

I have a list of the areas of "genius" for every one of my staff members, which allows me to quickly assign tasks to the right person.

Top of Your Game

The title of Daniel Priestley's book, *Oversubscribed*,[25] says it all. What would your business look like if you had so much business that you had to turn additional business away? That's when you could raise your fees substantially and only take higher-valued, higher-paying customers.

Here are some rules of thumb for attaining the nirvana of being oversubscribed:

Supply and Demand

1. Your business is worth a high value to a small number of people.
2. Demand and cost of your service or product becomes high when there are more buyers than sellers—it's as simple as that.
3. Demand for what you're selling must be high for you to attain high profits.

Become Your Own Market Brand

1. You don't need a massive market to be oversubscribed; you just need more people than you can handle.
2. It takes up to fifteen times for someone to get your message, so what are you doing on a repeated basis to get that message across?
3. You need to be relevant. Update social media accounts regularly so those who follow you have new content on an ongoing basis.
4. Collaborate with others. It's another opportunity to expand your reach.

---

25 Priestley, Daniel (2020). *Oversubscribed*. Capstone.

Four Drivers for a Market in Balance

1. **Innovation:** create something unique.
2. **Relationships:** build powerful relationships so that those people and businesses only want to deal with you. If you become an expert in your field, you'll be known as an influencer, and this will help you own the relationship.
3. **Convenience:** easiest delivery—for example, one-stop-shopping dentistry.
4. **Price:** there's an imbalance when what your clients need exceeds your ability to supply, which allows you to raise your fees.

A Single Player Per Niche

1. Most of us can't be what everyone needs *and* be the best at a specific thing at the same time. Innovation, for example, takes time to scale and costs money.
2. B to C (business to consumer): people don't want to buy what others are selling. They want to buy what others are *buying* (in other words, people are influenced heavily by advertising and promotions).
3. B to B (business to business): businesses mostly buy what they need.
4. People buy mainly because of their wants, not their needs. Find out what they want and package it along with their needs.

Buck the Trend

1. There's a good reason the collectibles industry is worth billions—people love to have items that are one of a kind. What does it take in your industry to be one of a kind?

Value Is Created in the Ecosystem

1. Develop a positive ecosystem that delivers a great service and has people coming back for more.
2. Give away information freely while charging for implementation. Consider all the options for losing weight. You could buy a book for $20, buy a gym membership for $500 a year, or hire a personal trainer for $3,000 a year—or you could get liposuction at $15,000. Your business needs to offer all the solutions from start to finish.
3. Innovation is important, but not at the risk of losing your winning formula. LEGO makes the same bricks they made decades ago. They may add new designs to the collection, such as special characters, but they continue making the same bricks.

Nothing Beats Being Phenomenally Remarkable

1. Replace your marketing budget with a *remarkable* budget.
2. How can you be the best in your niche?

I invite you to read *Oversubscribed* for yourself and carefully ponder how you can launch your business into an oversubscribed state. Sometimes, it takes challenging what we believe possible to uncover true potential—and, in turn, success.

GOALS

Gaining Traction

Gino Wickman has over twenty years of experience helping entrepreneurs gain traction and control within their businesses after successfully turning his own family business around. His book *Traction*[26] has sold more than a million copies, and his clients see an average annual revenue increase of around 18 percent.

He does this with a focus on systems, values, vision, organization, and entrepreneurial operating systems (EOSs).

According to Wickman, there are six components to any organization:

1. **Vision:** where are you going, and how will you get there? The more clearly your staff sees your vision—including for marketing—the more likely you are to achieve it.
2. **People:** surround yourself with the right people in the right seats.
3. **Data scorecard:** the best managers evaluate their staff and business through a set of matrices that remove bias, personality, and subjective feelings, leaving only the "What's So" of people. This data also empowers the leaders underneath you because by giving them a set of goals they can achieve, they know what's expected of them. For example, my office manager might report that our goal was bringing in $250,000 for the month, but we missed the goal by $10,000. That is simple and clear. Just the facts.
4. **Issues:** there are only a few issues that will occur in your business, and the same ones tend to repeat. Tracking this enables you to forecast the future.
5. **Process:** doing your business correctly allows for scalability and efficiency.
6. **Traction:** brings focus, accountability, and integrity to your business.

---

26 Wickman, Gino (2012). *Traction*. BenBella Books, Inc.

If you aren't happy with the current state of your business or your personal life, you basically have three choices: change it, live with it, or leave it.

Similar to what I have been sharing, the vision is crucial, as are the mission and core values. "People" is one of the three **Essential Pillars**.

The data scorecard comes in most handy in the Prosperity pillar. Issues, process, and traction are the "how to" in getting things moving in your business. EOS has trainers you can hire to help hold you to account for the growth that you want.

Let's say you have a goal of getting fifty new clients a month, and you get only forty. You look at your three choices: lower your expectations and live with a new, lower goal; try again for the goal; or abandon the goal entirely.

If you are committed to hitting that goal, then look at what is missing, which, had it been present, would have made a difference. It might be that you need to make 250 calls a month instead of 200, for example. Go back to my delightful funnel drawing. How many inputs—such as business calls—do you need to make to have the desired result come out the other end? It is as simple as effort in, results out.

Eleven Ways to Make and Attain Better Goals

How are your goals coming along? Here is my takeaway on that from Hal Elrod's book *The Miracle Morning* to help you:[27]

1. Make conscious choices that align with your values and propel you to your financial and emotional goals.
2. Evaluate the risks associated with those choices.

---

27   Elrod, Hal (2012). *The Miracle Morning*. BenBella Books.

3. Consciously choose a vision that encompasses a greater good.
4. Make choices that give your clients more value than they would get with your competitors. Use surveys to ask your clients regularly what their needs and wishes are, as well as where the problems are with you, your staff, and the services you provide. If you know the top three areas of concern, you can focus on those and deliver a higher level of service.
5. Ensure that your team is aligned with your vision and has all the tools to ensure you hit your goals, paying special attention to the customer experience—which starts with your website and your staff answering the phones, all the way to how and when the customer receives a bill and completes their experience with your business.
6. With laser focus, evaluate all aspects of your life that are important to you within each of the **Essential Pillars**, ensuring that what is most important has actionable items and that you start ticking them off.
7. Have a standard operating policy (SOP) manual like the one they use at McDonald's. Your manual should articulate every aspect of your business.
8. Set aside time not just for the "doing" of the business but for other aspects that support it, including marketing, returning phone calls, and responding to emails.
9. Keep the pipeline full, feeding it when it runs low so there's a steady stream of qualified leads coming into the business.
10. Have your finger on the pulse of your business. Know your statistics and reward the staff with bonuses. Fast-action results give the business momentum and hasten success.

11. Diversify. Look at related businesses, totally different businesses, and anything you enjoy that may result in income. Using the Four Investment Buckets (business, real estate, stocks, and investments), ask yourself, "How can I be in each one?" and, "How can I replicate success in each one, again and again?"

Now, let's take an honest look at the relationship we have with our habits and how those habits are either helping or hindering us in reaching our goals.

Goals and Habits

Anything you do repeatedly forms a habit, so it's important to ensure that it helps establish and advance your goals.

In a 1979 Harvard Business School MBA study on goal setting,[28] the graduating class was asked a single question about their future: have you set down your goals in writing and created a plan for attaining them? Here were the dismal results:

1. Eighty-four percent of the class hadn't set any goals whatsoever.
2. Thirteen percent of the class had written goals but had no concrete plans for achieving them.
3. Three percent of the class had both written goals and concrete plans.

In a follow-up ten years later, the 13 percent who had set written goals but no strategy were making twice as much money

---

28   Savara, Sid. "Why 3% of Harvard MBAs Make Ten Times as Much as the Other 97% Combined." https://sidsavara.com/why-3-of-harvard-mbas-make-ten-times-as-much-as-the-other-97-combined/.

as the 84 percent who had no goals at all. However, the three percent who had both written goals *and* plans of action to achieve them were making *ten times* as much as everyone else combined!

Why? Was it just because they made a plan?

No. Plans don't complete themselves simply by existing. It was the strong habits backing up those plans that motivated the former MBA students to follow through to the end, whereas the reward for lack of focus and discipline is often failure.

Remember, nonspecific movement and activity are not sufficient for major achievement. Taking positive steps that build on and move your game forward is required to produce stellar results.

I have many routines that I rarely, if ever, break—and it's all because I heard of that Harvard study and wanted only to be in the successful 3 percent. I always wake up at 5:30 a.m. (except for those rare occasions when I "sleep in" until 6 a.m.). I always spend two to three hours preparing for the day, which includes a Jacuzzi for thirty to sixty minutes to soften my muscles (multiple surgeries have left scar tissue, and I've had my share of physical limitations; the hot water helps me to function). I use this time to read my email and check my finances, being careful not to let my phone or iPad fall into the Jacuzzi and electrocute me.

I play for "email zero," meaning my inbox has *no* more messages. There are only three options when you get an email or a task: delegate, reply, or defer, and I try to do one of the three to everything in my inbox in this morning window. It is crucial not to have emails and social media eat up your valuable time.

I then hit the gym for forty-five to sixty minutes before finishing up in the sauna, where I sweat to detox while I meditate. I wasn't always so diligent, but I'm glad that's the person I've become. I understand that not everyone has access to a sauna and Jacuzzi—so you need to devise the systems and tools you need to win within the pillar of health.

PROSPERITY EXERCISE 5:
Habit Formation

Grab a piece of paper or open a blank document on your preferred device and answer the following questions:

1. What new habits are you committing to incorporate into your life that align with your values and will support your existing or newly conceived business?
2. What are the risks of these habits, if any, and what are the risks if you do not start these habits?
3. What is your vision of how these habits will work for you and support your existing or newly conceived goal?
4. What benefits do these new habits have for your customers?
5. Is your team aligned with your vision? Do they all have the same answer if you ask them, "What is the vision of our business?"
6. What is the one thing you can do today that can increase sales, profitability, and the customer experience? (I ask myself this question every morning and know what I will be focused on that day before I even get to the office.)
7. Is your SOP manual accessible to every employee? Does it need to be updated?

8. Do you have time put aside to work *on* your business—a dedicated time to return calls and emails and to contemplate what works and what doesn't—not just *in* it? It's not enough to have "CEO time" only when there's a lull in business. I strongly suggest you work on your business when you are away from the office.

9. What's your marketing plan? How will you track your return on investment (ROI)? Remember, the aim is a return that is at least 3x the amount invested for marketing.

10. What are your stats (if your business is already open)? What percentage is going toward profit, payroll, fixed and variable costs, and salary for you or for the person you delegate to run the business?

11. What percentage of your investments is diversified into each of the Four Investment Buckets?

TAKEAWAYS FROM THE PROSPERITY PILLAR

Rate yourself on your Prosperity pillar on a scale from one to ten. Do you know your numbers? Are you living paycheck to paycheck? Do you have money left over, or are you playing the game of shuffling money around to pay the bills? Do you have 3x your burn rate in savings? Is there money being put aside for investment? Is there any passive income?

Although there are formulas and theories about various percentages of your income to invest and numerous places to invest them in, in the end, it all comes down to the habit and behavior of consistently taking money off the top of your income before you can spend it and put it into a vehicle that has the potential to make money. Making money has very little to do with intelligence and everything to do with your behavior, as explained in *The Psychology of Money* by Morgan Housel.[29]

Four places money can flow (Note: knowing this is crucial to attaining financial freedom):

1. Burn rate (your monthly nut, including discretionary expenses)
2. Taxes
3. Debt service
4. Investments

Knowing this is so important because once you understand that there are only four places money can flow, you realize you either need to increase your income, decrease your burn rate, get better tax-saving advice, or pay off your debt so you can invest. If you don't invest, then you will toil for the rest of your life. Either you work for money, or you invest to have your money work for money.

Four buckets to invest in (this alone has been the main reason for my financial success):

1. Business
2. Real estate
3. Securities (stocks and bonds)
4. Insurance products

---

29   Housel, Morgan (2020). *The Psychology of Money*. Harriman House.

And if you believe in diversification, I suggest you participate in all four buckets.

The Five Prosperity Exercises:

1. **Prosperity Exercise 1**, The What and Why: the reason "why" you are doing this is crucial to know.
2. **Prosperity Exercise 2**, The "What's So" Question: if you don't have your expenses and income recorded, and if they are not updated regularly, there is no possibility of experiencing a breakthrough in finances. What can you cut back on, perhaps temporarily, so that there is more money for paying off debt and investing? What new income can you generate, even if it means burning the candle for a little bit so that you can get your 3x into savings?
3. **Prosperity Exercise 3**, Pay Off Debt: get your 3x into savings, and once that payment is no longer going toward debt, put it in an investment bucket.
4. **Prosperity Exercise 4**, Visualize Failing Forward: play big. Play for passive income.
5. **Prosperity Exercise 5**, Habit Formation: put 10 percent monthly into an ETF, such as Vanguard's VOO fund, until you can buy real estate. Rinse and repeat. Is it time to increase savings from 3x to 4x? Is it time to buy the next investment property? All of this is based on your goals and your sources of income.

Pillar 2
PEOPLE

1. **Prosperity:** revenue, business, economics, money, financial affairs, income
2. **People:** relationships, communications, rapport, family, significant others, personal friends, and business colleagues
3. **Personal:** well-being, welfare, self-worth, self-help, growth and development, mental and physical health, meditation, exercise, nutrition, time alone, spirituality, purpose and vision, happiness

WHAT BARBRA STREISAND SANG

People who need people are the luckiest people!
—Bob Merrill and Jule Styne

Barbra Streisand was certainly onto something when she sang that song. Studies show that infants who lack human touch and cuddling fail to thrive. People who are isolated fall into pits of despair. Both Japan and the UK have appointed a Minister of Loneliness, and other countries will no doubt follow suit.

People are the "why" of prosperity. Without social and emotional connections to those around you, you cannot progress in life, both from a personal and business perspective. Things fall apart. Mental health goes screwy.

Society is composed of people. People do things with us and for us. People provide a sense of community, friendship, and love that no technology, artificial intelligence, or stuffed animal can give you. People are important because they watch your back, set you straight, pull together as a team, and help each other out.

Relationships, including business relationships, are the foundation of your overall success. Without open communication with those who are important to you and without strong relationships, the other pillars wither and offer little, if any, value.

Let me share something a bit shocking: dentists make four times the average income and are highly intelligent—yet, they often abuse drugs and are twice as depressed as the general population. Why?

I believe it is because they learn on their way to the top to shed themselves of the people around them. And you know what Barbra Streisand would say to *that*.

To get into dental school, you must be at the top of the class, which typically makes you a lone wolf. You are *not* collaborating with others, and you're focused on cutthroat competition because you need to excel. By now, you have limited the number of friends in your circle if you haven't already turned downright antisocial. You are intent on doing life "by yourself," and, to top it off, most patients don't even want to be in your office because dental work can be scary and painful. Dentists are often on track to junk their People pillar, and it takes them quite a while to discover they're stuck with a two-legged stool—if they ever realize it at all.

Realizing this at an early age, I started to look at how I could be happy, social, and funny, and how I could make dentistry fun, enjoyable, and not painful. I made that my mission and shared it with staff and patients. I managed to build a successful and fun environment that most patients want to visit because they typically have a non-painful experience and leave feeling inspired. If I had simply become a snarling misanthrope, I wouldn't have any people around me—and no patients, either.

Consider the business world. You need people inside and out for a business to function. You need employees and management to keep the operations running. You need vendors who supply you with products or materials. You need customers who want what you offer and are willing to pay for it.

The employees of a company influence how well your business does through their skills, hard work, and creativity. Even a business with all the right plans is nothing without the people who enact those plans and see them through.

Also, humans are social creatures. In our private lives, we rely on our interactions with others. When you need help making a decision or you need someone's shoulder to cry on, you call on your people. Even going online to learn something new is only possible because other people have offered their experience to the world.

Nothing in life is truly accomplished in a vacuum. Like most people, I cherish alone time, but I also crave relationships—and relationships need work, beginning with clear communication.

COMMUNICATION IS KEY

Are you a human being? Yes? Great to hear! In that case, it may interest you to know that communication breakdown is one of the primary reasons that businesses, relationships, and just about everything else involving human beings falls apart. Wars take place because of communication breakdowns, and many marriages fail for the same reason.

Communication is the process of sending and receiving information—whether spoken, written, or nonverbal—and in today's world, we need it more than ever. It helps us connect with others socially. It helps us understand each other's wants, needs, and desires. Without it, the path to your pillars is steep and rocky.

Communication comes into play on some level every day with just about anyone you encounter—clients, vendors, co-workers, employees, spouses, partners, and loved ones, right down to the letter carrier. Without some skill in how to navigate the conversation, no business or relationship can thrive—in other words, the waiter you upset today may spit in your soup tomorrow.

There are three essential components to communication, which I like to call RIG: **Responsibility**, **Integrity**, and **Generosity**. This relates to all forms of communication, including verbal, text, email, and smoke signals. These three components are opportunities to be powerful and free in your communication.

In conversation, you are responsible for what you say and what you do *not* say. You are also responsible for what you hear and what you do *not* hear. This is the "clear" part of "clear and effective communication."

Ask yourself this question: Where does communication live—in the speaker or the listener? I believe it lives in the listener. Here is an example: Many of us may have attended events where the speaker was mumbling or their speech didn't quite make sense. Yes, they are speaking, but no one is listening, and no one is moved to follow the advice given. Remember this when you speak, and ask yourself: how can I speak in a way that will have someone listen? If you have RIG on your mind, you might find your message has a better chance of being delivered.

Responsibility in communication deals with owning what falls out of your mouth and acknowledging how the other person hears it. Some people don't give a flying fig about how their words land on other people's ears, but even if you didn't mean to scald them with an ill-conceived joke, for example, it doesn't mean you should walk away from the encounter annoyed at others for "not having a sense of humor." Empathy is required for clear and effective communication.

Many times, I have responded to someone's speaking with a solution, which is very "alpha-male reactionary." What I am taking on this year is pausing, allowing the other person to fully speak, and then responding with: are you looking for a solution (a practical answer), a hug (an emotional response), or do you want to just be heard (a social response)? I first read this in a *New York Times* article[30] and then heard it on multiple podcasts, and I think that this is the tool for me going forward.

On to Integrity, the "I" in RIG. The Merriam-Webster dictionary defines *integrity* as "firm adherence to a code of especially moral or artistic values."[31] I believe integrity boils down to doing what you say you are going to do within the time frame you promised. And, if the time frame or commitment changes, it means immediately getting into communication with the other party to obtain *their* agreement to the new time frame or content.

What, you wonder, does that have to do with conversation?

---

30 *New York Times* (2023). When Someone You Love Is Upset, Ask This One Question. *New York Times*. https://www.nytimes.com/2023/04/07/well/emotions-support-relationships.html.
31 Merriam Webster Dictionary (n.d.). *Merriam-Webster Dictionary*. Definition of "Integrity." https://www.merriam-webster.com/dictionary/integrity.

Here's an example of a conversation that lacks integrity going off the rails. One of you does not do something within the time frame the two of you have established. No matter how lovely and rewarding the initial conversation was, the person who does not make good on promises has undercut whatever power the interchange had and curdled it into a bad memory. Instead of bringing clarity, trust, and promise, this has sown distrust.

As for the "G" in RIG, Generosity, how do you bring that into dialogue with someone? You allow the other person to get their thoughts out without undue interruption. You hear what they say and also what they are trying to say, the unspoken subtext. You generously turn the spotlight on them and help them fill in their own blanks.

Considering how vital this is, everyone should put "improve communication skills" on their to-do list. I believe that if we all embraced the concept of RIG, there would be significantly more peace in the world and within ourselves, and we'd all be much more productive.

Public Speaking

There are many ways to become a better communicator beyond the usual one-on-one interactions. There are in-person and online courses and workshops. There are self-help books. There are also talk and behavioral therapies, which can help you work past whatever mental roadblocks interfere with your ability to communicate well.

Delivering lectures is another excellent way to become more comfortable and efficient with communication, as it forces you to interact with a large group and be on your toes when you answer their questions. For those of you suffering from a fear of public speaking, there are techniques for overcoming that fear, including getting into the kind of practice that lecturing provides. It gets easier, I promise. One of the reasons I have held three professorships is my desire to expand myself in the arena of public speaking. What better way to become an effective speaker than lecturing before hundreds of people?

If you're really sweating bullets up there at the lectern, just remember that you are offering your listeners the *gift* of your thoughts and knowledge. Your listeners do not care in the slightest whether you're having a good hair day or if there's a bit of lint on your jacket lapel, or whether you really look as young as you claim to be on that dating website. They only care about what you have to say.

According to research, the number one phobia is public speaking, followed by the number two fear—death.[32] It's amazing to me that some people would rather die than speak in public!

As a teenager, I was one of those people. In high school, I was completely terrified of public speaking, but when I realized story-telling and public speaking would allow me to share my feelings and ideas more easily—and help me in my future career—I began studying it and promised to stick with it. Later, I took leadership positions in youth programs, joined networking organizations, and took on major roles that required me to speak to groups often.

From there, as aforementioned, I began to lecture. I put myself in uncomfortable positions of having to do research and summarize it for students in a way they could absorb.

---

32 National Social Anxiety Center, (n.d.). "Public Speaking Anxiety"
    https://nationalsocialanxietycenter.com/social-anxiety/public-speaking-anxiety/

As I learned in a Landmark Education course,[33] communication lives with the *listener*, not the speaker. If you don't have someone's attention—if you're speaking into a void—then your speaking is ineffective. The art of effective communication is to *enroll* the listener to hear what you're saying.

One technique I picked up is to start a university class with a dictionary definition of "lecture," followed by a slide with my own personal definition: being talked to death. The audience usually chuckles. I further get their attention by offering Starbucks gift cards to anyone who engages me in meaningful dialogue.

And guess what? The lecture happens! People engage, and no one feels talked to death. There's a powerful, palpable level of active listening. This concept of lecturing, teaching, and public speaking does not take away from the crucial aspect of looking inward and working on your flaws, challenges, and fears. It is not sufficient to develop a strong public speaking muscle without developing the ability to love, empathize, and relate to others.

As a dentist, my fingers are in people's mouths most of the time, which makes dialogue tricky and monologue an art—and a requirement. When I'm on the stand as an expert witness for dental malpractice and dental injury cases, being comfortable in front of a judge and jury is essential. I have testified or reviewed more than a thousand expert cases over the past three decades and relied on my training and continuous expansion in speaking nationwide to build confidence and ease when it comes to public speaking. Public speaking can be a needed skill if you are in business when it comes to articulating your point of view or product. It can help you get more clients and network. It can make you known as an expert in your field.

---

33 Landmark. (n.d.). *Landmark*. https://www.landmarkworldwide.com/.

The pinnacle of my dental career occurred in my fifties when I received notice from my alma mater that they were giving me an award for the work I had done in my nonprofit, Homeless Not Toothless. The award would be given at Madison Square Garden in front of 10,000 people! And would you mind giving the keynote speech to the graduating class while you are there? I imagined what my English teacher would have thought if she were still alive, sitting in the audience. I went from being criticized in her 10th grade English class as someone who would never amount to anything to giving a talk at the number three dental school in the country about the over 135,000 people we have helped receive over $11 million in free dental care. To date, the honor of giving the commencement speech at NYU was the highlight of my dental career.

Don't Just Hear—Listen

Like most people, I am capable of talking a blue streak, but it is just as important to learn how to be a good listener.

Listening is an often-overlooked skill, but it can make the difference between a good and bad conversation. The best listeners are those who don't just hear what people say but understand the other's intent. To do that, you have to peel back the onion layers. It takes knowing that we all just want to be "heard"; we need to listen to others without rushing to understand, fix, or change them. Often, when we listen intently, that is all we need to do.

Anyone can *hear* what's said, but not everyone *listens*. Not everyone picks up on the hidden truth, the subtext, the ideas people are struggling to get across. Not everyone has a silver tongue; most people misspeak. They meander. They overuse filler words. Not everyone was the darling of their high school debate club, but if you listen well, you can still decipher their private, coded messages, and they will love you for it.

One way to become a better listener is to stay present—*truly* present, not giving-it-lip-service present. It involves staying mindful of the person you're with and tuning in to their needs and emotions. It involves reading their body language and interpreting their tone. It's not hurrying to talk and fill the silence.

Listening well means making eye contact, not interrupting, and taking notes if needed. It means being able to paraphrase what others say and ask questions when necessary. It means being open to hearing what others say (even if they're not saying it the way you want to hear it) and being able to understand the essence of what they're trying to communicate, even if you don't agree with them.

What matters is ensuring that your conversation partner knows you are putting in the effort to listen and engage in a deep way. The reward is when the other person says, "I feel heard."

Tell Me a Story

Storytelling is a type of public speaking. It is a fantastic tool for getting people's attention, helping people relate to each other, and learning about untried experiences.

To tell a good story, you don't just need something to tell; you also need the confidence to tell it. If you mumble and stumble, it becomes awkward for you and for the listener, and it closes off the possibility of immersion.

If you want to have an impact on the people around you, improve your public speaking skills. Mastering it has been one of the secrets to my success and has allowed me to communicate comfortably with celebrities and billionaires and to enroll people into doing business with me.

If you are one of the many who fear public speaking more than death, I strongly recommend getting past this by taking online or in-person classes on public speaking and storytelling. Practice in front of increasingly large groups. Seek therapy if the fear is entrenched.

Do whatever you need to do to achieve mastery in this area. Your success—whether describing your business or telling a special someone how deeply you care—depends on you becoming comfortable with yourself and not being fearful or shy.

In *Purple Cow*, Seth Godin writes about what you need to do to differentiate yourself from the competition—to be a purple cow, not a typical black-and-white one.[34] Communication is a great tool that can bring you to the top of the charts. I believe this is one of the main reasons that no one has ever sued me. It is rare for a medical practitioner to escape such an occurrence; thus far, however, I have been spared.

My website is updated regularly, and I ensure there are clear communications throughout. For example, I post a page that gives patients free advice on products I recommend—products I do not sell or make a commission on. Empowering patients to care for themselves without trying to upsell them builds trust and sets my business apart from those who hawk the products from which they profit, regardless of quality.

Love Languages

The term "love language" was first introduced by author and counselor Dr. Gary Chapman, whose books break down five primary love languages:[35]

---

34 Godin, Seth (1997). *Purple Cow*. Penguin Random House.
35 Chapman, Gary (1988). *The 5 Love Languages*. Northfield Publishing.

1. **Words of affirmation:** genuine compliments and praise.
2. **Quality time:** giving undivided attention.
3. **Gifts:** giving and receiving thoughtful presents.
4. **Acts of service:** performing acts or services that make others feel loved and appreciated.
5. **Physical touch:** a back rub, hand-holding, hugging, any kind of nonintrusive physical connection that offers comfort.

Have you ever tried to connect with someone but later worried that the way you went about it was somehow wrong? Clunky? Tin-eared? Or, at the very least, ineffective?

Understanding how people feel loved and appreciated is vital in forming stronger bonds. If a friend's preferred love language is quality time but you hardly see them, don't give them a box of chocolates in hopes that it will suffice. Someone who wants most of all to spend time with you does not want a gift card or an item from a store, even if it's handmade, as thoughtful as such a gift might be. They can get their own snow globe or pair of gloves anywhere; that's not what speaks to them. A gewgaw in a box will not make them feel as loved and appreciated as sharing an afternoon lemonade on the porch. Instead of a happy glow, you'll wind up with a flickering disconnect between the two of you.

Be careful, too, about giving versus receiving. There are benefits to both, but do not confuse how either act will make *you* feel. Put the feelings of the *other* person before yourself. You will naturally benefit in the process as well.

Even in business, knowing what makes your employees and clients feel appreciated makes a world of difference to them. People want to feel like *people*, not numbers, and using the right love language is a great way to accomplish that.

I've asked my staff which of these languages speak to them and made note of it. This way, when it's time to praise them for a job well done, I check their love language first and respond using the same language. If they like words of praise, I don't shower them with bonbons.

My wife points out that the more people become aware, the more they speak more than one love language. The healthiest relationships recognize that their partners dance between different needs and wants and often have multiple love languages.

PEOPLE WHO NEED PEOPLE

One of my "superpowers" is a photographic memory. Once I realized that I could see detailed pictures in my head and recall them years later, I used this to my advantage.

As an undergrad, for example, I tape-recorded seminars, took copious notes, reviewed the recordings to ensure the notes were accurate, and then transcribed my notes onto the blackboard in the very room where I would later take the test. When it was time for the real thing, I could recall the "picture" of my notes on the board. This helped me complete undergrad in only two years and gain acceptance into my number one choice for dental school—NYU College of Dentistry.

You would think that with a superpower like a photographic memory, dental school was a cakewalk. You would be wrong!

I was on academic probation for the entire first year. As a nineteen-year-old, the youngest in my class, I felt honored to be in a medical program at all—but I felt as lost as a person could possibly be. I remember sitting in anatomy class with more than 150 other students when the secretary of the academic dean handed a note to the professor, who read it and announced to the class, "Would Jay Grossman please come to the front of the room?"

My classmates murmured about me being in trouble, and as I took the walk of shame to the front of the class, the secretary said, "Please come with me." I felt exactly as I did in 10th grade English class when the teacher said, "Grossman, you will never amount to anything." Those four words, "Please come with me," can never mean anything good.

"Well, Dr. Grossman," said the academic dean as I shrank in my chair. "It looks like you're having some struggles."

She was right. My GPA was below fifty, and I was getting Fs in my classes. Saying I was having "some struggles" was an understatement. I could hear Mrs. Killjoy in my head all over again: "Grossman, you will never amount to anything."

I explained to the dean that I was up eighteen hours a day, seventeen of them in the library, but it wasn't helping.

"How about a tutor?" she asked.

"I don't have the money for that," I replied, "and I walk alone."

"We cannot let someone for whom we waived two years of undergrad fail, and you need help," she said, "and this idea that you are doing it by yourself—you can forget about that entirely."

I used to think I needed to cross the finish line all by myself, or my victory wouldn't be worthwhile. Having help seemed like something only cheaters did—or, at least, I felt help was only for those who really needed help, and I was above that. Looking back at my astonishing naïveté, I can see that I didn't yet realize the value of mentors and partners. I didn't have any in my business life until I was in my forties. Perhaps it was luck or persistence or both that kept me in the game despite missing such important players on my business team.

When the dean of academic affairs suggested getting a mentor, I was not yet at the point in my life where I understood the value of teamwork or getting help, but neither did I want to get kicked out of school, so I sucked up my pride and called the person she recommended—and who the school was gracious enough to pay on my behalf.

If it wasn't for Dean Fuss and the backing of NYU College of Dentistry, who noticed my struggles, and if it wasn't for Dr. Paul Lanza, the upperclassman who took me under his wing and taught me the science of medicine, I wouldn't be a doctor today. Mrs. Killjoy once upon a time messed with my head, but she wasn't the only adult whose voice mattered in my life.

I do not have sufficient words to express my gratitude to my many mentors—those who supported me, believed in me, and gave me an opportunity to grow and learn. I'm grateful I was able to say yes to something I normally wouldn't have and thus able to put the concept of "doing it alone" behind me.

With a Little Help from Your Friends

Published in 1936, Dale Carnegie's revolutionary self-help book *How to Win Friends and Influence People*[36] has sold more than thirty million copies worldwide, making it one of the best-selling books of all time.

A book written nearly a century ago remains relevant in the modern age by understanding the fundamental principles of people. Using these principles regularly and turning them into habits will do wonders for your connections with the people around you, both in business and in your personal life.

Carnegie divides his book into numerous fundamental principles. Here are my favorites:

---

36   Carnegie, Dale (1936). *How to Win Friends and Influence People*. Simon & Schuster.

Don't criticize, condemn, or complain. Andrew Carnegie and Charles Schwab never criticized people, and that's why they had the same loyal employees working for them for decades. Sharp criticism of others often ends in futility. Instead of condemning people, try to figure out what makes them tick. Figuring out this means you are coming from love, as you are committed to learning what has made someone do or say something as opposed to jumping in and criticizing them.

Give honest, sincere appreciation. Bait the hook to suit the fish. If you are literally going fishing, a worm on the hook works better than a strawberry, even if you personally love strawberries. To influence people, give them what *they* want, not what *you* want. If you make others believe you are feeding their underlying desires and really care about them and their success, they will work well for you.

I have someone on my payroll whose main job is to gather the goals, dreams, and aspirations of my staff and put a game plan together to ensure their success. That's a big part of why the culture in my dental office is strong, with very little turnover. Several staff members choose not to participate in this, which is fine, as it's their choice—although I would like to think they will realize in time that when you have goals, and when you have someone holding you accountable for them, those goals are more likely to come to fruition.

The best way to succeed is to see the situation from the other person's point of view. Even during negotiations, consider writing a pro and con list from the other side's perspective. How can each party gain from the negotiation? If this is the premise on which you build, you'll end up with a win-win.

People learn best from praise, so make sure you're liberal with it. Thank others for their efforts, compliment outstanding traits, and ensure the praise is specific and personal to the individual.

Make the other person feel important by expressing genuine appreciation and respect. Comments like, "I'm so sorry to trouble you, but can you please ..." go a long way. When someone does something nice for you, regardless of whether you requested it, offering a simple "thank you" gratifies them, and it also makes them more likely to help you again in the future.

Become genuinely interested in other people. The most common word in conversation is the pronoun "I," says Carnegie. People tend to talk about themselves more than anything else, which is not the best way for *you* to win friends and influence people. The best way is to be interested in the other person—which is, of course, that person's favorite topic! Focus on helping others impress *you* instead of you trying to impress *them*.

Speak with them about their achievements and dreams, and invest time and energy in them as professionals and people. Convey to others your interest by doing things for them—spending time with them, perhaps spending money on something that will support their goals, celebrating birthdays, and being selfless. Even consider your tone of voice when you answer the phone: try to convey a welcoming interest. When you're interested in others, they become interested in you.

Smile.
Remember names.
Be a good listener.
Consider and be sympathetic to other opinions, ideas, and desires.
Welcome disagreement.
Don't fight.
Don't say, "You're wrong."
Admit mistakes.
Friendliness is the way.

Yes. Get the other person to say "yes" as often as possible at the beginning of a conversation.

Let people think it was *their* idea. The best way to get people to do something is to make it so they want to do it themselves. That's how Mark Twain's Tom Sawyer got every kid on the block to take a turn whitewashing that fence for him. They even gave him something in return for the privilege of getting to do his chores.

In my dentistry practice, I ask people for their ideas on what they want, such as what they would like to see their teeth look like. From that, I formulate a treatment plan that stems from their wants, needs, and desires while still being governed by my professional expertise. Making what you do feel like it's the other person's idea is sometimes difficult but important.

Walk around in their shoes.

Appeal to nobler motives.

Dramatize results, but don't be a drama queen.

Throw down a challenge.

Simmer down.

Don't be bossy.

Consider egos.

Thank your opponent.

Get on the same page.

Summary:

- You do not have to live your life or run your business alone. The most successful people know the benefits of mentors and understand the value of delegation.
- When you're interested in others, they become interested in you.

- The first step in keeping disagreements from becoming arguments is to acknowledge them, recreate what the other person's position is, and ensure you understand their point of view.
- Start the conversation with the things you have in common.

Using People Without "Using" Them

Allow me to frighten you for a moment.

You may think that if you have a significant other and maybe a good friend or two, you're done working on your People pillar. After all, business is business and has nothing to do with this pillar, right?

Wrong.

Here's just a sampling of the areas involved in running a successful business:

Staffing, human resources, inventory, vendors, leases on office space and equipment, salaries and taxes, office culture, marketing, statistics, revenue, production, quality assurance, checklist of responsibilities, standard operating procedures, marketing leads, following up with customers and clients, clearing incoming emails, responding to voice messages and missed calls, bank account balances, online reviews and responses, quality assurance of your product, keeping the office clean and presentable and smelling nice, ensuring supplies are stocked, reordering and checking that the supply price is not inflated, checking bank balances daily, public relations, collection calls, acknowledging birthdays, returning calls, lease negotiation, IT support and equipment, architectural design, instruction on how to use and maintain equipment, bank loans and terms, marketing and messaging, training staff, analyzing statistics, monitoring line items in terms of meeting or beating industry standards, understanding profit and loss statements, understanding cash flow, understanding balance sheets ... hold on, I need another coffee!

If this partial list has changed your mind about opening, running, or investing in a business, that was not my intention. The point is that most people simply cannot and should not manage *all* these puzzle pieces on their own. In fact, most businesses do not account for all of those crucial aspects of running a business. Perhaps that is why 50 percent of small businesses fail in the first five years.

They say you should always use other people's money (OPM) where possible. In the same vein, you should always use others' skills to ensure you can tackle all the components of a business with confidence.

For this, you need people. And if your People pillar is crumbling to dust, that's a problem.

Although you do need to master a few of the above areas of expertise if you're running a business, this is really where your staff and consultants come into play. Imagine trying to run a business without the proper team and systems in place—it's no wonder so many businesses struggle early on, especially when egos get in the way!

Igor and the Trunk

"Fine," you say. "But it's still business. Everyone in business is just a cog in the big ol' wheel, right?"

I'd like to slap your wrist for that. Instead, I will give you an example of what sounds like a business question but is really a People question:

How do you find a good insurance broker?

I don't know how others do it, but I'll tell you how I met mine.

Thirty-plus years ago, I attended a get-together for an emerging nonprofit organization. I arrived late, and the place was packed, so I sat near the back. Beside me sat a man who introduced himself as Igor. It's an uncommon enough name in California that it was easy to remember, but that isn't the only reason I recall the meeting.

Igor and I ventured into polite conversation. "Did you find a safe place to park?" he asked, as it was not the best of neighborhoods.

"I'm good," I said. "I trained in martial arts, and I keep a gun in the car for emergencies."

For some people, that response would have shut down the conversation. Not Igor.

"Hey, I've got a gun in my car too!" he said.

Later into the meeting, when we'd both had enough, we went out to the parking lot for a little show-and-tell.

Fortunately, our vehicles were parked close together, so we both popped our trunks to take a look at the goodies.

As we stood there examining each other's weapons, a thug approached us from behind with a knife. He must have noticed two men in good suits standing near pricey cars and reasonably assumed we would be easy targets.

"Give me your wallets," demanded the clueless thug.

When we wheeled around to face him, our show-and-tell guns still in our hands, the knife-wielding assailant dropped his knife, wet his pants, and bolted.

Without missing a beat, I turned to Igor and said, "I think we just bonded!"

It turned out that Igor[37] was an insurance salesman with an impressive portfolio, and I had recently considered getting into

---

37   PFR Advisors. (n.d.). *PFR Advisors.* https://www.pfradvisors.com/.

investments as the next stage of my financial diversification. Igor now helps me with my investments, the value of which just topped nine million—a nice hedge for retirement.

While I am not suggesting you go around discussing firearms with strangers, remember that a lot of surprising connections can come out of chance encounters—with *people*. Never take people for granted. For example, I had a best friend whose wife happened to be my wife's best friend, which made hanging out together, vacationing together, and seeing each other often easy and fun. Until, that is, there was a divorce. Based on the reasons for that breakup, I chose to no longer associate with my then-best friend. That difficult choice was based on integrity and love.

Trust: The Flight from Yemen

Now that you're winning friends and influencing people right and left, how do you keep those bonds tight?

One way is through mutual trust.

My friend Julie—an immigration attorney who has helped my family with personal legal challenges in the past—called me to ask a favor. After everything she'd already done for me, I immediately said yes.

"But this is a big favor," she said. "Don't you first want to know what I need?"

"No. I trust you, and I know you wouldn't ask me if it weren't important."

Julie explained there was a teenage girl in Yemen whose parents in the United States had just received citizenship here. The girl was very ill with stage four brain cancer and would likely die before having a chance to say goodbye to her loved ones. As a minor, she wasn't permitted to manage her oxygen machine on her own and could not get on a plane without it, but her family wasn't allowed to go to Yemen and personally escort her—this was during a time of harsh immigration policies during the Trump presidency.

Making things worse was that, although the mother had sued the administration and won citizenship for her children, the designation would only take effect while the kids were still under the age of eighteen—and the seventeen-year-old daughter's eighteenth birthday was looming fast.

Julie needed to fly to East Africa in two days to pick up the girl and fly her to the States, but she didn't have the medical training required to operate the oxygen machine. That's where the favor came in.

Before becoming a full-time dentist, I'd worked in my youth as an EMT and was a certified CPR instructor. I was medically qualified to escort the girl to the U.S. My family and I had a ski trip planned, but we all agreed that this took precedence, so we postponed our plans.

Two days later, Julie and I boarded many planes over the course of thirty-two hours to get to East Africa. We found the teenager in an ICU that did not resemble the kind of critical care we often take for granted in America. Doctors and nurses were swatting flies off the girl, who had already slipped into a coma. There wasn't much time left to reunite her with her parents for their final farewells, and I wasn't sure how we'd get permission for her to fly in her condition, but somehow, Julie managed to persuade the powers that be.

On the plane, I was in scrubs—which either made the other passengers feel more secure or more frightened. A first-class seat was the only space that could fit the comatose girl and the necessary medical equipment. I taped IV bags to the bulkheads and pushed thirty different drugs through the IV every few hours.

Then, mid-flight, the girl lost a pulse, and the oxygen tank failed because the AC power supplied to her seat wasn't working. To avoid an emergency landing, we used some of the extra oxygen supply kept on the plane for emergencies.

I began to resuscitate her, knowing that the chances of a spontaneous heartbeat were slim, and we still had over three hours before landing in Los Angeles.

Many aren't aware that CPR is not used to wake someone up by restarting their heart. Medically, CPR is designed to keep the blood flowing into the brain so that an advanced medical team can administer drugs and shock the heart—none of which was available to us at 35,000 feet. I would have to perform CPR for the remainder of the flight, all three hours of it. As I was performing CPR, the passenger behind me asked if I needed help. He identified himself as an anesthesiologist. I gratefully accepted help, and he confirmed there was no pulse, so I continued CPR.

The pilots came out of the cockpit and discussed making an emergency landing in Portland, thus missing our opportunity to bring her to Children's Hospital in Los Angeles. They said the protocol was to land immediately if someone onboard loses a pulse—but that's when the strangest thing happened.

Her heart started beating again.

It should not have been possible, but it was. Somehow, the young woman managed to survive the flight to Los Angeles. The pilots acquiesced to my request to land in Los Angeles, where we had a bed for her at a children's hospital.

The media naturally got involved. I summarized it thusly: two Jewish Americans flew to Africa to collect a Muslim child who was dying so she could see her Muslim family, who had recently got U.S. citizenship, one last time. She died at 35,000 feet, somehow came back to life through CPR alone, and was delivered to a children's hospital—on Christmas Eve, no less—where she managed to hang on for another thirty-five days.

No one can explain it, then or now. As an agnostic Jew, all I can say is, it was a Christmas miracle! The experience renewed my faith in the bonds among people to help each other and those in need. The experience of saving a life and bringing someone back from death is indescribable. I never thought that helping a friend fulfill her desire to help a client would result in one of the most impactful events of my life. My score on the People pillar for relationships with friends, travel, giving back, gratitude, love for work, risk, and excitement was a 10 out of 10 for many weeks. When I returned home, my children and wife were there to greet me. I was exhausted from being up for nearly five days with only catnaps and mentally fatigued from having someone die and come back to life on my watch. I wept in my wife's arms for what seemed hours. It was one of the most important events of my life.

Forgiveness: Don't Judge

What if you find you have misplaced your trust in someone? They screwed up, they stood you up, or they didn't come through. You're ready to cut the cord. Does everyone deserve a second chance?

The short answer is yes.

Take Felicity Huffman, one of the warmest, most genuine people I know. I see how she and her husband, William H. Macy, parent her two beautiful daughters. When the news broke of the college entrance exam cheating scandal, for which she eventually served eleven days in jail, I wrote an article coming to her defense—not to say that what she did was right, but to speak to how we all make mistakes, that many of us do extraordinary things to help our children, and that Felicity immediately admitted to wrongdoing and paid one hell of a price for it. "I accept the court's decision today without reservation," she said when sentenced. I admire that tremendously about her, and I am proud to call her a friend.

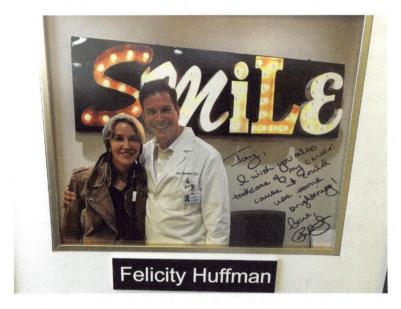

Felicity Huffman

Figure 5: Felicity Huffman and Dr. J

So, yes, everyone deserves a second chance. But the longer answer is that while everyone deserves a second chance, not all people allow themselves to rise to the opportunity of deserving one. If you close yourself off from the people around you, it shouldn't be a surprise if they, in turn, pull back.

What about people who have committed horrible crimes? Do you give them a second chance as well?

Try not to judge someone else's experiences. There are very few people in the world who are genuinely "bad." Most who commit crimes or abuse substances have reasons for their actions, even if you don't know or understand those reasons.

It doesn't mean their reasons are necessarily logical or sound, just that people often feel justified in their actions because of their own experiences. Many feel forced into paths leading to bad behaviors and can't find their way out, even if they would like to.

Would you want someone else judging some of *your* bad decisions? And don't tell me you've never made any!

Shazam!

Do not underestimate how much you need people and how much good you can accomplish with their help. That is how my nonprofit, Homeless Not Toothless (HNT),[38] came to be. HNT is my legacy.

I first met my future wife, Briar, in the dorms of NYU. We moved to California in 1989 and were only married a year when we had our first baby. I didn't have my California practicing license yet, so I decided to enlist in the Navy. They would accept my New York license—allowing me to practice as a military dentist—and offer benefits, so it was an obvious solution at the time.

I spent three years on military tour as a dental officer, from 1989 to 1991, and opened my private practice in West Los Angeles after exiting the Navy.

Because of my experiences, I immediately noticed people sitting on the side of the road near my office across from the VA Hospital in Los Angeles. They held signs begging for the kindness and generosity of passersby: "I'm a veteran, please help."

I started by giving a dollar here and there when I could, but I wasn't sure what use such small change could be and

---

38   HNT. (n.d.). *HNT*. http://www.hnt.dental/.

was concerned the money would go to drugs and alcohol. Eventually, I switched to offering them food, but I still didn't feel as if I was doing all that I could to make a difference.

One day, I reached into my wallet, and my hand closed over my business card. That's when the idea struck. I started telling those vets where to find my office, which was not too far down the road.

That was the glimmer of the idea for Homeless Not Toothless, which did not start out as a nonprofit—until I got a call from the Pentagon.

Let me set the background.

I was on active duty during the first Gulf War in 1990. I completed my tour of duty in 1991 and opened my private practice in Brentwood.

In 1992, the Pentagon called. I assumed I was being recalled, and all I could think about was running off to Canada. I had started my practice, I had enormous debt from it, I had two children still in diapers, and I was not ready to go back into the military.

"What do you think, Lieutenant?" said the colonel when he was done talking to me.

"Sir?" I asked. "Does this mean I'm being reactivated for military duty?"

"Did you hear a word of what I just said?" he barked.

"Sorry, no. Uh, sir."

He repeated himself, and this time I listened.

"Lieutenant, we've heard about the dental care you're providing to our veterans, and we would like to take your photo, place it in a ton of magazines, and make you the poster child for military recruitment. Are you interested?"

"Absolutely!" I said. "Oh, and by the way ... does this pay?"

Hey, it never hurts to ask! In this case, it did not hurt a bit—I told them Homeless Not Toothless was a nonprofit, and the military kicked in ten thousand dollars.

Technically, I didn't have a nonprofit. I had never filed for one. But with a ten-thousand-dollar contribution and built-in publicity, I immediately called my attorney.

"I want you to apply for nonprofit status today," I told him.

A few weeks later, a military photographer came to my office, and soon, my mug was plastered across the land in *TIME, Sports Illustrated, Better Homes & Gardens*, and nearly twenty other publications that together accounted for more than twenty million views.

Now we're talking!

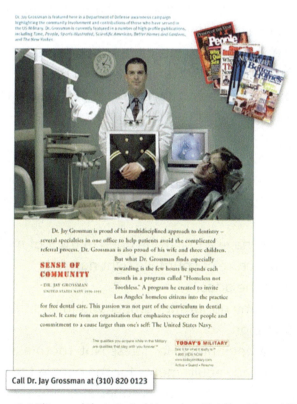

Figure 6: Military ad that started Homeless Not Toothless, 1991

"You've got my nonprofit number, right?" I asked my attorney. "So I can collect that ten thousand dollars?"

"Jay, it's only been three weeks," he said. "It could take a year."

"No, that's too late!" I sputtered. "I've got publicity, I've got seed money. I need that sucker now!"

I dialed the IRS. I was fully prepared to be on hold for a week—but lo and behold, someone picked up in only ten minutes!

"Ma'am," I began, "I'm sure every call you get is a problem, and I know you're just the messenger for a huge organization, and I wish I had something easy for you, but I'm in a world of hurt to get a nonprofit number. The military is recognizing me for the work I'm doing with veterans, and I have a vision of raising the pride and dignity of unhoused veterans through quality dental care. They are about to cut me a check for ten thousand dollars, *only* if I have nonprofit status."

To which she asked, "Sweetie, are you Dr. Grossman?"

I froze. Oh, no, I was on my way to debtor's prison in shackles! They had caught me at last! Or maybe it was a prank; I studied the ceiling for a hidden camera. It must be part of some hideous reality TV show.

"Yes, I'm Dr. Grossman," I said guardedly. If you lie to the IRS, they probably have a right to arrest you on the spot. "How did you know?"

"Because I have a magazine open in front of me, and I am looking at a picture of your face right now."

What are the odds?

I received my nonprofit number within less than a month of my application.

From the beginning, Homeless Not Toothless was not a free-for-all. I had requirements for the people I treated. They had to be at least ninety days sober and actively looking for work. The purpose of the free dental care was to empower them to get off the streets, which wouldn't be possible if they were still using drugs.

Today, Homeless Not Toothless is celebrating thirty-plus years and has treated well over 135,000 patients from all the collective clinics around the Los Angeles area, with services valued at over eleven million dollars (as of 2024).

We will discuss philanthropy in more detail later, but note how my philanthropic impulses would not have come to fruition in a bigger way had it not been for the help of people, often total strangers.

You want more people? I got 'em!

Bringing in celebrities to endorse a charity is a must. Celebrities have a reach well beyond what I alone am capable of, which is why I wrote nearly a thousand letters and sent them out cold, hoping for the best. Only one responded—and one is all it took.

Dorit Kemsley, fashion designer and television personality, called. She'd noticed Sharon Stone's name on the board of my nonprofit, something that was of interest to her since Sharon was her neighbor. Apparently, Sharon brought Dorit cookies the day she moved in, and ever since, Dorit had looked up to Sharon and followed her lead. Dorit, too, wanted to get involved in Homeless Not Toothless.

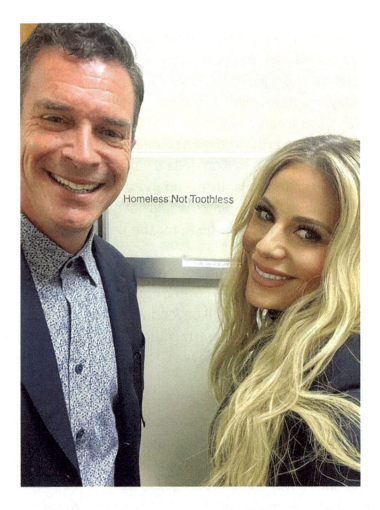

Figure 7: Dr. J and Dorit Kemsley of The Real Housewives of Beverly Hills, 2023

Shortly after our call, Dorit was on the game show *Beat Shazam*, hosted by Jamie Foxx, where she won $87,000 and publicly announced she would donate her winnings to Homeless Not Toothless.

When Jamie Foxx heard about the nonprofit from Dorit, he announced: "Let's round it up to a neat $100K!"

In 2023, Dorit called to set up another fundraiser for dental work for those in need. This time, the opportunity would put me on national television.

We filmed for three hours about Homeless Not Toothless, but because it was reality TV (*The Real Housewives of Beverly Hills*[39]), they used very little of the footage in the end, focusing instead on another part of my story—my fourteen kids! (Yup, you heard that number right; more about this at the end of the book.) I was initially disappointed by the decision not to discuss my nonprofit and focus on my personal life, but Dorit assured me it was nothing to worry about.

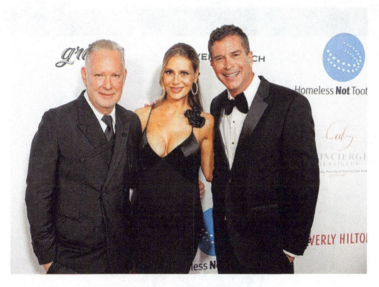

Figure 8: Homeless Not Toothless Gala; PK, Dorit and Dr J, 2023

She was right. Emails and donations have flooded in about Homeless Not Toothless ever since. We threw a gala in Beverly Hills that featured Paula Abdul, all of the *Real Housewives of*

---

39   Real Housewives of Beverly Hills. (n.d.). *The Real Housewives of Beverly Hills.* https://www.bravotv.com/the-real-housewives-of-beverly-hills.

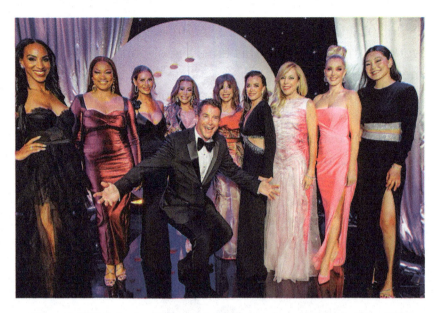

Figure 9: HNT Gala; Dr. J with the Real Housewives of Beverly Hills, *2023*

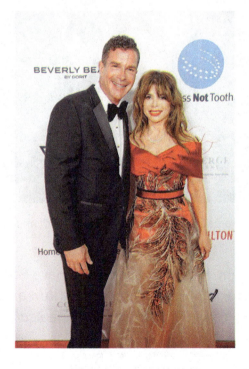

Figure 10: HNT Gala; Dr. J and Paula Abdul, 2023

That's right, it takes people. People who need ... well, you can take it from there. You know the lyrics.

Karma: Don't Judge a Book by Its Cover

Through Homeless Not Toothless, I was treating a man who was a few years older than I was. While working on his teeth, I mentioned to my assistant Jennifer that I was excited.

"I'm about to mix cement at my house," I said. "I've never done it, but hey—how hard can it be?"

I had plans to build a cement retaining wall along my property and thought that surely, with a medical degree, I could figure out how to whip up a batch of cement. After all, I do that every day—to glue crowns on top of teeth.

The patient raised his hand, something I ask my clients to do when they have something they need to say. I pulled my hands out of his mouth and allowed him to speak.

"Do you need help with the cement wall?" he asked, to my surprise. "It's trickier than you think."

I gave my address to a man I'd only just met, who had wandered into my practice from a local homeless clinic after completing six months in a residential sober living facility. Does that sound like a bad bet to you? On paper, perhaps. But in real life, I had a good feeling about this guy. Something in my gut told me to accept the man's generous offer.

John[40] showed up at my door promptly the next morning at 7 a.m., which is more astonishing than you may realize. I live in Malibu Hills, which is a winding, confusing area, and this was before the age of digital maps and GPS apps.

---

40   Homeless Not Toothless. (n.d.). John Brennan, Homeless Not Toothless patient. https://www.youtube.com/watch?v=Kgfs_177NgM&t=4s.

I showed John the project and the three bags of cement I had bought.

He looked around. "Where's the rest?"

"The rest of what? It's for a small wall."

"Three bags aren't enough," he said firmly. "What about the wood?"

"Wood?" I asked. "Perhaps you don't understand. This is for a wall of concrete."

John patiently explained that once mixed, concrete is a liquid, so planks of wood are necessary to prevent it from deforming and slipping while it hardens into the shape needed.

"Oh, of course," I said, trying to cover my ignorance and confusion. "Anything else?" Surely, there wouldn't be anything else.

"Rebar," said John.

"Uh-huh," I said, taking out a notepad as I realized I was already in way over my head. Clearly, I had no business monkeying with cement!

"Rebar helps hold the liquid concrete together," John explained helpfully.

"Rebar, right." I scribbled it down.

I didn't know John from Adam, but I handed him $500 to go get the supplies I had never considered getting.

Maybe other people in John's situation might have taken the money and run, but three hours later, he pulled up in an ancient station wagon with no shocks, the bumper dragging on the ground from the weight of the supplies. We were in business. The wall I thought would take me twenty minutes took both of us three days.

"How much do I owe you?" I asked John, once we had a beautiful new wall in place.

He looked insulted.

"You just gave me free dental work that cost a lot more than this," he said. "I'm tired of handouts. I'm happy to pay you back by working for you."

Impressed with John's professionalism and craftsmanship, my wife offered him another job, but only on the condition that he accept payment. He added a roof over the barbecue area.

After that, we kept him busy redoing each room of the house. He was always on time, always professional.

And then we invited him to live with us.

We did that after a police officer stopped by to tell us to watch out, that there had been recent reports of a guy living in a broken-down car. Malibu Hills is not an area where you see that kind of thing every day, and I realized that it must be John—and that he had nowhere to go.

It turned out that although he did have a place at a local shelter, he couldn't afford the gas to get there and back from working on our house every day.

At first, John didn't want to take us up on the offer, even though we had plenty of room. In the end, he stayed with us for two years.

In that time, I learned more about him. He had once owned a construction company, but his greed had gotten the best of him, along with substance abuse. Poor decisions had led to his wife and two-year-old son leaving. All that had taken place fifteen years prior.

His story was so sad, I couldn't leave it alone. I Googled his wife's name.

When I finally found his ex-wife—after making dozens of calls to dead-end numbers I had found online—I explained that John was nine months sober and living with us. That he was turning his life around and wanted to make amends. In his personal growth, he had managed to change his mindset, realizing that his wife had been right to leave him. He understood where he'd gone wrong and genuinely yearned to apologize for his mistakes.

John's son was by now finishing high school and had a summer free. I arranged in secret, with his mother's permission, of course, to fly the kid out from the Midwest and have John drive to the airport "to pick up a visitor."

It was a reunion I will never forget. Taylor, his son, ended up staying with us the entire summer. He and John were able to build a strong bond despite all their years apart.

A few years ago, twenty years after John first helped me, he shared with me that he'd become successful enough again to reward himself with his dream—a Harley motorcycle, something that might not have ever been possible for him if I hadn't mentioned building a simple wall the day I had worked on his teeth. I flew out to New Mexico where John was now living, rented a motorcycle, and he and I spent the good part of a week playing like we were in *Wild Hogs*.

And, to my way of thinking, if I hadn't thought of starting Homeless Not Toothless, I wouldn't have had the opportunity to see how one kindness leads to another and how these little ripples of kindness can turn entire lives around.

John's story does not end there.

One night, while he was still living with my family and me, he mentioned something odd.

"Working with you sometimes reminds me of working for celebrities," he said.

I thought he was joking, especially when he name-dropped Sharon Stone and her sister, Kelly. I thought nothing more of it until a few weeks later when I got a call on my cell from someone saying she was Sharon Stone.

"Right," I said.

"No, really."

"Sure. And I'm the King of Albania."

"It's fucking Sharon Stone!" she snapped.

That was all I needed to hear. The delivery was too on-point to be fake.

"But how did you get my number?" I asked, which was only one of many questions swirling in my addled brain.

"From John," she said.

"Oh, okay," I said, although how and why John Travolta had my number to begin with, and why he would give it to the star of *Basic Instinct*, I couldn't figure out.

"Yes, John's sister used to date my assistant, and they're still in touch," she said. "That's how I learned about your work with veterans and adults who are struggling."

Only then did I realize that John Travolta didn't have a sister who dated women—but "my" John did!

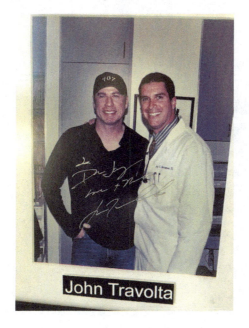

Figure 11: John Travolta and Dr. J

"I'm wondering if you'd be interested in expanding your work to foster kids," said Sharon. The administration of then California governor Arnold Schwarzenegger had recently pulled dental coverage from foster care services.

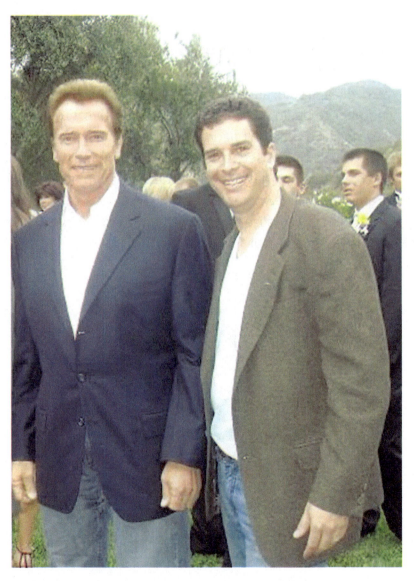

Figure 12: Arnold Schwarzenegger and Dr. J

A few days later, after chewing over Sharon's idea, I heard that The Terminator himself was, coincidentally, in my dental building. The opportunity was too perfect to miss, so I had my assistant handle the office while I rushed to the lobby to catch Arnold on his way out.

I muscled my way past his security detail (okay, I didn't *literally* muscle my way past them, but I boldly approached) and gave Arnold a quick explanation of what I wanted to meet with him about. I ended by saying, "How does an ordinary person like me, who wants to make an extraordinary difference in society, get your attention for a few minutes?" With that, he granted me an audience the following week at his house, which was not far from my office.

During that meeting, the first thing I said was, "Why on Earth would you take dental care out of the supported foster care service?" Perhaps I used somewhat gentler terms. I mean, the guy is still buff.

Arnold explained that the State of California was broke. They had to cut something. It occurred to me that those in foster care were too young to vote, so they probably weren't high on the list of people the governor needed to court.

I left there pretty disheartened, not just because of his decision but also because I'd helped vote him into power. But when I called Sharon to tell her what had happened, she was undeterred.

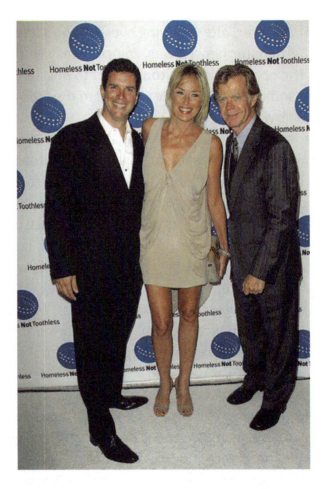

Figure 13: First HNT Gala; Dr. J, Sharon Stone, and William H. Macy

"Let's get a meeting with the director of Family Services," she said. "I'll set up a lunch."

I never thought I'd hear such a sentence from Sharon Stone—not directed at me, anyway. I was further surprised when she attended the meeting in person alongside me.

What the director, Dr. Charlie Sophy, told us was quite sobering. Apparently, many schools would not accept foster children without proper dental examinations, which put a lot of the children at a further disadvantage—and there were around 30,000 of them in foster care at the time.

Think about it: you take kids away from parents who are abusive, incarcerated, or dead, and then you deprive them of an education because they can't afford a dental exam? Mind-boggling. What type of person in this position will be emancipated into society at age eighteen?

I suggested we raise funds and attention with a gala. Sharon agreed to be the guest of honor. I dug into my client base and asked Bill Macy to host, and other celebrities—including Larry King—turned out, as well.

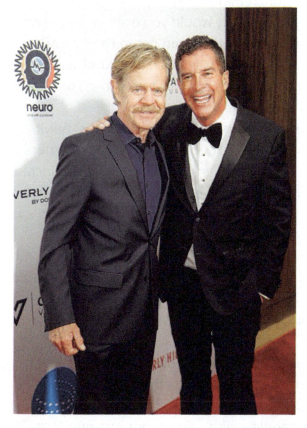

Figure 14: HNT Gala 2023; William H. Macy and Dr. J

From that start, we were able to build several clinics which now see ten to fifteen thousand children each year. As of 2022, we have treated more than 135,000 homeless veterans, foster children, women in domestic abuse situations, and the poor, offering free dental services valued at over eleven million dollars' worth of dental care as of 2024.

Today, Sharon is a board member of Homeless Not Toothless, and I am thrilled to call her a friend. All these good things came from the humblest of networking opportunities through a once-homeless dental patient named John, who had friends in high places.

John's story reminds us that you wouldn't want someone to mistreat you—so why would you ever mistreat someone else? Sometimes our emotions can get in the way of remembering the golden rule, especially when the world seems to be against us on a given day. It's okay to make mistakes. You're human, and mistakes are how you learn.

It's important not to hang onto the habit of ignoring or insulting those around us. It alienates others and has a negative impact on everyone's mental health, including yours. Personally, I have learned to steer clear of those who are not kind. My time is too precious to allow others to spatter their poison onto me.

When you treat others with love and kindness, they're more likely to do the same in return and pass it along to others as well.

Kindness and Caring: Bill Macy

The government issues us our Social Security ID number for use in employment and health care. Maybe that encourages some people to see others as faceless entities, but in truth, we're all people—with names, not just numbers. That is why it's important to ensure you recognize those around you as full human beings, even if they're not your *favorite* human beings.

They're not a number; they're not an "it." They are people who were once sweet little babies deserving of love and care, just like you and me.

You can't plan on where you're going in life—your goals, your vision—until you're clear about who you are being. "Being" is the state of being real, being your authentic self, and not hiding behind a façade designed to make you look good. It's about who you are when no one else is looking. It's your "real" self. Your fake self might pretend to show a caring side, but do you have a caring side when you are exactly who you really are?

I'll bet you do.

Now, ask yourself what drives you to care about others. Is it about the way it makes you feel when you do something good for them? Is it about the benefit you receive from engaging in an act of kindness? Is it because you've been in someone else's shoes before and can empathize?

There is no right or wrong answer. It's what you make of those reasons, how you use them to channel your motivations and actions, and how you treat the people you help that matters.

It's okay to feel good about helping someone else. It's okay if that feeling drives you to continue helping others, as long as you offer genuine kindness and compassion and not just a kindness placebo to rack up another do-gooder notch on your belt.

Listen to others and give them the help they need, not the help you feel like giving or think they deserve. Do it for whatever reasons you do it, but do it with sincerity.

One of my favorite actors is William H. Macy—not just for his roles in *Fargo, Wild Hogs,* and *Shameless,* but for who he is as a person. He came into my practice some twenty years ago when another actor referred him to me for his dental care. I felt honored, and my admiration only grew as I basked in the glow of his friendship and marveled at his willingness to help me in two profound ways: helping to grow Homeless Not Toothless, and assisting my youngest son, Ari, in getting an acting education.

When Sharon Stone and I decided to have a gala to raise funds for Homeless Not Toothless, Bill was an immediate "yes" to serving as emcee. On a personal note, I also asked Bill to look at a two-minute monologue my high-schooler son, Ari, had acted in. Bill watched the monologue and asked me to call Ari, who picked up the phone and said, "Hi, Dad."

"This is not your dad; this is Bill Macy," the star told my son. "I just saw your monologue, and you have the bones to become a great actor. Go get an education, and let's do a movie together."

Bill and his wife, actress Felicity Huffman, were kind enough to have Ari and me over for a coaching session before Ari attended acting school in New York.

These are the untold stories the public doesn't know about actors: the human side, the kind side, the nonpublic side. Actors, idols, sports figures—so many of them are quietly helping people they don't know without sending out a press release to soak up public love and sympathy. I hope Bill doesn't throttle me for shining a spotlight on his private kindness.

Briar Puts Her Foot Down

Remember how I said I overheard money arguments between my parents when I was growing up and decided the answer to all that was to grow up to earn as much money as I humanly could? And how I thought that if my father had only worked at a big job that was farther from home, he'd have more money, and therefore, all the troubles of the world would come to an end?

Well.

Fast-forward to my marriage, five or ten years into it. As I mentioned earlier in this book, there was my beloved wife, ready to pack her bags and leave me.

I was floored. Briar and I had had our ups and downs over the years, as in any relationship, but I did not see this coming. Wasn't I being a good provider?

"You're not *available*," she said.

It stung.

This was my wake-up moment when I realized that Prosperity was not the only pillar I needed to master. I was financially successful, yes, but it came at the cost of working ninety hours per week. I began to see my wife's point: we barely saw each other.

Briar's ultimatum shocked me into realizing my mistaken belief that providing money was the most important thing in a family. I needed to fix this; my marriage depended on it. I went on to find a better work-life balance and have done my best ever since to stick to it.

My wife, fortunately, is very strong in the People and Personal pillars, while I am strongest in the Prosperity pillar. We balance each other out. That probably has a lot to do with why we're still happily married after thirty-seven years and counting.

PEOPLE EXERCISE 1:
Size Up Relationships

Rate your important relationships on a scale from zero to ten. Overall, what number do you give yourself? Do you consider your communication with these people

effective, emotional, and trusting? Give it a score,[41] with zero being ineffective, without emotion, and non-trusting, and ten being the exact opposite.

Ask those people on your important relationships list what *their* views are of the relationship you two have. What score would they give it, using the same criteria? It will be interesting to note if your score is similar to the ones others give you!

PEOPLE EXERCISE 2:
Size Up Communication Skills

Rate yourself from zero to ten on your ability to communicate, your comfort with public speaking, and your ability to resolve conflicts.[42] Are you reactionary and angry? Are you calm and committed to a resolution? Give yourself a score, with zero being ineffective and ten being extremely effective.

Keep track of this score, preferably on the same spreadsheet as your finances—you can add a tab to the same sheet—and put a date and score on the page. Update it weekly. Just as in the prosperity section where we discuss measuring and reporting as crucial, the same holds true in the personal pillar. Tracking communication skills is just as important as tracking financial scores.

---

41   Dr. Jay Grossman. (n.d.). ***Essential Pillars*** *People Exercise 1, Size up Relationships.* https://www.drjaydds.com/.

42   Dr. Jay Grossman. (n.d.). ***Essential Pillars*** *People Exercise 2, Communication Skills.* https://www.drjaydds.com/

That which is measured improves. That which is measured and reported improves exponentially.

—Karl Pearson

Essential Pillars People Exercise 1, Size up relationships

as of	TODAY()		
Relationships Index, Score 0 - low, 10 - hi			
	My communication with my significant other is effective		
	My emotional connection with my sig. other		Sig Other
	My trust in my significant other		
	My communication with my family is effective		
	My emotional connection with my family		Family
	My trust in my family		
	My communication with my staff/co-workers is effective		
	My emotional connection with my staff/co-workers		Work
	My trust in my staff co-workers		
	My communication with my friends is effective		
	My emotional connection with my friends		Friends
	My trust in my friends		
	Other relationships that are important enter here		

#DIV/0! Average Score, Relationships

TAKEAWAYS FROM THE PEOPLE PILLAR

The People pillar demands excellent communication skills, emotional connections, and strong relationships. How do you rate yourself in this pillar, on a zero to ten scale?

There are three essential components to communication:

Responsibility: Own up to what you say and do not say.
Integrity: Do what you say you are going to do, within the time frame you promised, and re-promise if you need to change the time frame.

Generosity: Be generous in listening to others instead of hogging the spotlight.

Questions to ask yourself:

- What steps are you taking to improve your communication skills?
- What are your love languages, and what are your significant other's love languages; are you fluent in each other's love languages?
- Are you clear on the steps of how to win friends and influence people?
- What will be your legacy to your loved ones?

Pillar 3

PERSONAL

1. **Prosperity:** revenue, business, economics, money, financial affairs, income
2. **People:** relationships, communications, rapport, family, significant others, personal friends, and business colleagues
3. **Personal:** well-being, welfare, self-worth, self-help, growth and development, mental and physical health, meditation, exercise, nutrition, time alone, spirituality, purpose and vision, happiness

GETTING UP CLOSE AND PERSONAL

"Personal" is everything that goes into keeping the mind, body, and soul healthy and capable.

When you require **physical strength**, you work out and eat well.

When you desire **mental strength**, you read and research, get therapy or coaching, and expand your knowledge and understanding.

When you feel a lack of **spiritual strength**, you break away from the world and spend time in reverence, introspection, and possibly worship. Or you join others in celebration. Find out what works for you, what makes you feel good, and what gives you the personal rejuvenation that the body and mind need.

All these activities fall under the umbrella of the Personal pillar, and all are vital to achieving complete health and wellness, inside and out. When you rate yourself on a scale of zero to ten, factor in career choice, health, nutrition, exercise, recreation and vacations, the environment at home and work, happiness, contentment, hobbies, risk tolerance, excitement, chill time, how you give back, and your gratitude, all these factors contribute to your Personal pillar.

Of these habits, nutrition, lifestyle, and exercise make up the largest percentage of the key success factors for this pillar. You can have awesome workouts, but if you eat like crap, sleep haphazardly, burn the candle at both ends, and muddle through poor relationships, this pillar will crumble to dust.

Happiness is something you define, and if you are seeking happiness by itself, it often leads to depression and sadness if there is no meaning or purpose in your life. Happiness comes from belonging and being accepted for exactly who you are, which is why the People pillar is crucial to the well-being of the Personal pillar. Once you find relationships with people who love and accept you as you are, and you have meaning and purpose in your life, happiness follows organically.

The Case for Health and Wellness

Just the way a business cannot operate without functioning components, human beings cannot sustain themselves without seeing to their own needs. Success in long-term health and wellness springs not from doubling down on work or amassing more greenbacks, but in understanding the interplay between exercise, behavior, nutrition, and overall wellness.

Internal: Mental and spiritual health are the first things most people think of when referring to internal health, but physical wellness likewise has an internal focus. What you eat and drink may hit your stomach first, but it breaks down into what does and does not nourish the whole body. What you eat affects your organs and bodily functions—as well as your mood. Essentially, anything that occurs within the confines of the body counts as internal health.

External: Mental and spiritual health also has an external aspect. People around you can be quick to notice the results of exercise, especially if you've gone after a rippling six-pack—but your inner attitude and behaviors also affect your external experience. Everything we say and do plays a part in the physical world around us; in turn, we can either benefit or harm the health and wellness of others.

With the external in mind, let's first break down some aspects of physical health.

EXERCISE

So, exercise. Does it really matter?

Yes. Case dismissed.

Okay, the longer answer is that if you can get your body up and active to some degree every day, that's ultimately what matters.

It would take all my cloud storage to make an exhaustive list for you of all the benefits of exercise. Health, morale, self-love, better sleep and cognitive function, lower blood pressure, higher energy—I think you know the drill. Whatever your situation, accept it, deal with the issue, and work on improving it. In this sense, health is no different from business. You need to identify the weaknesses and build them up with systems, routines, and self-monitoring to help you improve them.

Do I hear a few groans out there? Drop and give me ten!

Exercise does not necessarily mean getting a pricey gym membership, pouring yourself into Lycra, and pumping iron until you pass out. Exercise comes in many forms, including simply doing more of the things you love—such as walking, hiking in a beautiful spot, gardening, or splashing in the pool. Even something as simple as stretching counts toward exercise goals, because it gets your body moving and keeps your joints limber. Stretching is also a great way to stay physically and mentally relaxed.

Similarly, breaking a sweat doing pretty much anything counts toward a cardio workout. You can break a sweat from swimming (although you won't necessarily realize it), doing housework, walking briskly from the car park, dancing wildly in the privacy of your living room, or pushing your kids on the swings.

Exercise is about living fully inside your body. It's about treating your body with love. As long as you get moving, your body will thank you.

Estimates are that more than half the world's population will be overweight or obese by the year 2035—that's four billion people who don't look good in Lycra, not just you! (Actually, *no one* looks good in Lycra, so you are definitely not alone.)

With obesity rates on the rise, let's take action to break this trend. Buddy up with a friend or family member and exercise together to keep each other accountable. By doing this, you'll be supporting your People pillar as well as your Personal pillar.

*Early to bed, early to rise, work
like hell, and fertilize.*[43]

—*The Wealthy Gardener,* by John Soforic

Soforic's work is all about fertilizing your life, investments, and relationships. If you are not constantly working on watering and pruning, you'll get stuck with weeds. He extends the analogy of tending a garden to encompass building wealth, health, and happy relationships. Exercise provides clarity of mind, increases cognition, boosts energy, reduces stress, focuses the mind, and bolsters your ability to withstand shocks, setbacks, and breakdowns.

Edward Smith-Stanley said those who do not find time for exercise will have to find time for illness.

Finding the Right Fitness Routine

My youngest son, Ari, is a personal trainer who works out ten times a week when he's competing. Building and maintaining that kind of endurance doesn't come easy to many people. Not to mention, he was a very overweight child. When he transformed his body to compete in 2023, I could not be prouder of what he had had to do to become this sculptured!

---

43 Soforic, John (2020). *The Wealthy Gardener.* Penguin Random House.

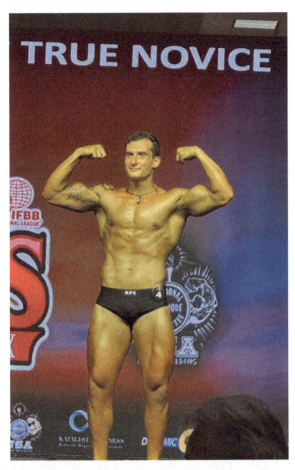

*Figure 15: Dr Jay's youngest son Ari, competing
after being an overweight adolescent*

Did I say, "Endurance doesn't come easy to many people?" I meant *me*. It has never come easy to *me*. I wasn't a jock in my youth, and when I did participate in sports, I had to work at it. Then, when I was forty-seven, some irreparable damage was done to my body. Although I was fortunate to receive excellent medical care, when I was confronted with these post-accident injuries, I had to work hard to get through my frustrations, limitations, and pain.

Physical fitness is individual, and you need to take that into account. Each person's metabolism is different. Some people can lose weight just by walking twenty minutes a day and naturally have great flexibility and stellar bloodwork. Others must work harder at it.

Age, gender, genetics, current health, past history—it all matters. Always check with your doctor before embarking on any new health kick, and gradually build up to what works for you and what doesn't.

The thing is, if you start out with a fitness plan you detest, you're not going to follow it. Often, what stops people from engaging in a consistent exercise routine isn't laziness; it's that they can't seem to find a routine that suits them.

Just as every person is unique, there is no one routine that works for everyone. It can take active time and effort (and sometimes a dash of cash) to find what works best for you. It's a process that can quickly become frustrating, especially with so many techniques, gurus, and gadgets at your disposal.

How do you find the routine with your name on it? The same way Goldilocks found the perfect bowl of porridge: by testing the options.

No one is stopping you from committing to a more intense workout routine—but don't assume it has to be at a gym, or with a personal trainer, or with specialized equipment. You'd be amazed at how much household furniture and items can tone and shape you. Examples include push-ups against the windowsill, deep knee bends with your tush barely grazing the sofa, calf raises on the bottom step of the stairs, and bicep curls with soup cans. There is an army of fitness experts with their own YouTube channels, many of them demonstrating standing workouts that only take a few minutes and don't even require a mat.

The problem lies not in having too few or too many choices, but in trying and discarding those choices too quickly before you've really had a chance to test them. By rushing things, you may not have the chance to make the adjustments that otherwise would have totally worked for you.

Instead, try approaching this the way you'd approach the Four Investment Buckets—one at a time, with patience. Give yourself at least a few weeks with one system to see if it fits.

Schedule five or ten minutes out of your day to pause and give a promising routine a try.

Baby steps can lead to healthy cardiovascular leaps.

Tools for Success

Have you ever tried to stand up after sitting for a long period, only to find your muscles and joints creaking and complaining? That's a sign you've been inactive for too long. At least stretch some of those aches out. Better yet, take a short walk around your living room or office.

Me? I follow a ninety-minute rule. I never sit for more than that length of time, be it writing this book or in everyday life. After ninety minutes, I always break off and take a walk, or even just pace around a bit, to distract my mind and body for ten to fifteen minutes. Then I come back to my task, right as rain. This helps me rejuvenate and prevents, or at least decreases, fatigue.

If you're one of those people who looks up to discover with alarm that night has fallen and you haven't even gotten up to eat, set a timer to remind yourself to stretch and move around.

Remember, you can use ordinary household objects to help you achieve certain fitness goals. I prefer a wider approach; here are some of the products and services I use to help me achieve my health and wellness goals:

1. **GADGETS:** mine include a Fitbit to monitor steps; an Oura Ring for 24/7 heart rate monitoring, personalized health insights, and sleep analysis; and a WHOOP band with real-time coaching that helps me train smarter, sleep better, and recover faster.
2. **COACHES:** for exercise, relationships, business, nutrition, and mental health.
3. **INFORMATION:** I read at least two books a month on self-development, business, or other subjects that otherwise support the areas where I am weakest.

Motivate Yourself, Don't Force Yourself

Remember when you were a child and your caregivers woke you up earlier than you wanted to because you had to go to school? You probably griped and groaned and struggled to shuffle out of bed, even if you'd had a full night's sleep.

Why?

Because you were being forced to do something instead of motivating yourself to do it willingly.

Let's face it, some annoying things in life are necessary—like getting up on time for school or work. But if you can figure out how to motivate yourself, even the most annoying tasks can become that much more enjoyable, or at least bearable. The question is, how can you drum up motivation when it seems to come and go of its own accord?

Train yourself.

Pick something that *does* motivate you. Perhaps it's a favorite (healthy) snack or a guilty pleasure such as a television show, with which you can reward yourself after completing an exercise routine. Eventually, you'll start associating the enjoyment of your reward with the completion of your task.

My geometry teacher in tenth grade was cool—he wore a bolo and knew how to teach and motivate. He had a particular way of letting everyone know how you did on a test, as he handed back the graded tests in ascending order. This means that if you were the first to get your test handed back, it was the lowest grade, and if you were the last to get your test handed back, it was the highest grade.

Well, sometime about a minute or so before he was done handing back tests, Myra would start chanting, "I'm getting the last test, I'm getting the last test." It did not matter that she was right; everyone hated her! (It turns out she graduated as valedictorian.) Regardless, it was infuriating, and I took this on as a challenge—beating Myra became my motivation. Now for a bit of background: the final counted for 50 percent of your final grade, and if you chose to retake the test, your new grade would be the average of the two tests. Those were the rules. So, it came to the final, and Myra was ahead of me by one point. I got a 96 on the final; she got a 98, and I needed a 99 to beat her, so … I showed up for the retest.

The teacher said, "What are you doing here?"

I replied, "I'm going to beat Myra!"

I further stated my dilemma, which was even if I got 100 on the test, that would give me a 98, which would tie her—so I offered the following new deal: if I got 100, he would round up my grade to a 99. If I got a lower grade, so be it; my final grade would go down. Well, you know what happened—otherwise, I would not be writing this paragraph. I literally had classmates outside the room cheering me on, and Myra was yelling and screaming, "It wasn't fair; the rules changed after the fact." Well, Myra, now that it is forty years later, I admit that you are right. It wasn't fair to change the rules after the fact. That said, thank you for being my motivation to excel, to do better. My A+ in math helped me with financials later in life, so I am very grateful.

There are two things to keep in mind here—one is to be mindful of just how much you're rewarding yourself, especially if food is your motivator. Don't reward yourself with a fatty feast just because you got your butt in gear for five minutes.

Secondly, at least until your exercise habit really sticks, only use those specific rewards for this specific activity. Don't go popping the popcorn every time you do something else, or you may gravitate to the activity you consider slightly less onerous. If you watch an episode of *Real Housewives* every time you wash a dish, you'll have sparkling dinnerware, but you'll have lost the connection between real exercise and that particular reward.

Time Management

Too short on time to do a single sit-up?

In *The One Thing*, authors Gary Keller and Jay Papasan discuss how Jerry Seinfeld uses this technique with tremendous results.

Skeptical? Me too! Fortunately, I happen to know Jerry, so I asked him if this was accurate. Jerry confirmed that he blocks out 8 a.m. to noon every day for uninterrupted time to develop his comedy. He celebrates at noon with a variety of options that he always looks forward to as a reward for the morning's hard work. Since his passion is cars, he often takes one of the many vehicles in his collection out for a spin.

There's a lot of wisdom in this. Jerry puts time aside *first thing in the day,* which produces a result that gets an immediate reward.

I developed a similar routine for myself, based on my own body clock and my likes and dislikes. I wake at 5:30 a.m. most days and immediately ask myself, "What is the one thing I must do today to move the ball down the court?" (An activity which, let me note, would also be very aerobic if I weren't simply using it as an analogy.)

I then expand my question: "What is the one thing in each pillar I must do today to grow and better myself?" I follow this up with time blocking to ensure there's a span devoted to each pillar.

My last pillar of the day is to review the next day's schedule and plan for it to go as smoothly as possible. I set my phone alarm ten minutes prior to all major appointments scheduled for the next day as a safety check to ensure I run on time and keep my word as it relates to specifically scheduled calls or events.

Success and failure all come from your schedule. You can forecast someone's success or failure by looking at what they have or have not planned. This is a screenshot of my calendar program to show how I use time blocking to ensure I am participating in each of the **Essential Pillars**.

6 AM	6-7 PERSONAL PI...
7 AM	7-8:30 PERSONAL PILLAR. Time Bloc...
8:30 AM	8:30-11 PROSPERITY PILLAR. Time Block: Expert Work/DDS, TAG - game is to...
11 AM	11-noon PROSPE...
12 PM	NOON - PERSONA...
1 PM	1-5 PROSPERITY PILLAR; DDS, expert, TAG, Real Estate
6 PM	6-8 PEOPLE PILLAR Time Block: Dinner / Family time 2 hrs
8 PM	8-10: PERSONAL PILLAR Time Block: complete the day,...

Starting at 6 a.m. (the latest) is a big block of time dedicated mostly to my Personal pillar. I hop into the Jacuzzi to get my body parts moving. I balance my finances, evaluate stocks, and reply to emails. Then it's exercise, meditation, and sauna.

On to my Prosperity pillar, recalibrating my financial goals and checking up on any of the business tasks on my plate at the moment.

At noon, I'm back to the Personal pillar, taking care of myself, rewarding myself for my morning accomplishments, and giving my brain a rest.

Next, a big chunk of time for my Prosperity pillar, generating new business or working on existing projects from 1–5 p.m. Working on the business, not just 'in" the business. I prefer to do this away from the office, so I am not sidetracked by the everyday distractions.

By 6 p.m., I turn into a people person, enjoying dinner and family time for a couple hours before finishing off the night tending to my Personal pillar again from 8 to 10 p.m., when I prep for the next day. I look at the next day's schedule and set alarms on my phone, ten minutes prior to each important event for the following day, to keep me on track.

DIET

Diet isn't just about how much you weigh or whether you look as skinny as an influencer on TikTok. What we put into our bodies is what fuels us each day, which is why it's important to be mindful of what we consume.

We've all heard the axiom, "You are what you eat." Well, it's true—although, perhaps not in the way you think. Unhealthy eating decisions can lead to increases in body fat, sure, but what you put in your mouth also travels around your system and affects every part of the territory—which is to say, your body and your brain. We are what we assimilate (what the body absorbs), which is why I believe in functional medicine and having your blood and stool checked at least annually to see what is working and what is not functioning at its best.

Eat well, and you're likely to feel physically and mentally energized. Eat junk food all the time, and you'll feel crappy. Feeling crappy leads to thinking crappy thoughts, and crappy thoughts chip away at your mental health. Garbage in, garbage out!

Can You Hack It?

I'm not a nutritionist, but here are some common-sense hacks for finding a better way to nourish yourself:

Digestion Hack: Stomach acids break down the food you eat and extract the valuable components, so don't dilute their awesome power by bloating up on liquids before or during your meals. If you're drinking all that liquid in an attempt to curb your appetite, make non-creamy, vegetable-centric soups a recurring part of your meal plan; at least they offer nutritional value while curbing your appetite.

Also, take a gentle stroll—what was known in stuffier times as a postprandial walk—for at least twelve to fifteen minutes after large meals, without *getting* your heart rate up. It helps stabilize blood sugar and keeps you from the dreaded after-dinner drowsies.

Nutrition Hack: Eat the main course first so enzymes fully extract the valuable components of your food. Do what Europeans do by having your salad next, which is also a good time to introduce liquids.

I often pass up dessert and have an appetizer instead as a final course, if I'm still hungry, but you don't have to banish sweets and salty snacks from your life forever. Banning them often leads to feelings of deprivation, which just boomerangs you back into even worse eating behavior, so allow yourself treats in moderation. The "moderation" part isn't just another way to punish you, by the way—the less you pickle your body in sweets and carbs, the faster you lose those cravings. Your "pain" will be short-lived.

Alcohol Hack: At a party, instead of having everyone rag on you about not pouring alcohol down your gullet until you cave and order a double, order soda water with a lime wedge. It will pass as an alcoholic drink, and you won't have to explain your choices or put up with peer pressure.

"Eating" Your Stress

Not all stress is bad.

You read that right! In the TED Talk "How to Make Stress Your Friend," Dr. Kelly McGonigal discusses the difference between good and bad stress.[44] Stress and anxiety, which leads to the

---

44 McGonigal, Kelly (2013, June 1). "How to Make Stress Your Friend" [Video]. TED Talk. https://www.ted.com/talks/kelly_mcgonigal_how_to_make_stress_your_friend?subtitle=en.

fight-or-flight instinct, isn't an automatic sign that something is wrong. It's your body's way of preparing you to handle a situation or task, and that can be a *good* thing.

There is a temptation to run to the snack drawer every time you feel a bit of stress coming on. Fat, sugar, and carbs can provide (very) temporary comfort, but this is usually not helpful in the long term.

No one wants to be in a constant state of stress, but understanding the difference between the good and bad kind can help improve your overall health and wellness while increasing confidence in your ability to handle challenging situations without resorting to plunging into a food coma for relief.

Working hard for something or someone we don't care about is bad stress. Working hard for something or someone we love can cause stress, sure, but we easily recategorize it as passion and excitement—and those feelings are *motivators* as opposed to *demotivators*. Those are the stress vibes that can lead to positive change.

As we alter our perception of stress and when to embrace it as a friend, its wear and tear on our hearts lessens.

Reading Diet Books

Books are a form of consumption, too, and it's one of the easiest ways to "feed" the mind. Fiction, nonfiction, biography, fantasy ... whatever your preference, the written word does amazing things to the brain, and that goes as well for listening to the written word with books on tape. Just think how far humanity has come in ways of sharing knowledge and imagination.

If your brain is hungry, check out the list of some of my favorite books in the Additional Reading section at the end of this book.

Spirituality and Religion

Even if you're agnostic or an atheist, spirituality is yours for the asking.

For some, it's about a specific deity or belief system or book of scriptures. For others, it's about energy and vibrations. Just about everybody has experienced that overwhelming feeling of being one with this marvelous universe of ours.

Spirituality can be whatever you want it to be, and it is an important component of the Personal pillar—and of simply being human.

There is no right or wrong when it comes to spirituality, beyond being able to find comfort and peace. It can be about nature and animals. Silence and rest. Vastness and the wonders of the tiniest atomic particle.

It can be about tapping into your thoughts and feelings on a deeper level through meditation or yoga. Embracing the teachings of a master. Finding your own way or following an enlightened path.

Where or what is your mental and emotional happy place? It truly is important to find the place, inside or outside, that reliably makes you happy—be it a physical location, a religious tradition, or a sacred rite performed alone or with others.

I have a sacred rite of my own. I schedule time with my guy friends for a scotch or to go dirt biking. This is what reliably brings me happiness and provides a necessary break from the daily routine.

Philanthropy

At face value, "philanthropy" probably brings to mind grand acts and huge sums of money that can change the world at large.

True, but there's so much more that goes into the concept of philanthropy. You don't have to wait until you're a billionaire to participate.

You know by now that I love dictionaries, so here's what Merriam-Webster has to say about *philanthropy:* "goodwill to fellow members of the human race," "an act or gift done or made for humanitarian purposes," or "an organization distributing or supported by funds set aside for humanitarian purposes."[45]

I am not suggesting you start up a humanitarian organization—although, if you want to, you have my blessings—but note how humanitarian kindnesses can include the smallest act, such as buying coffee for a police officer who's stuck outside in the winter directing traffic.

I was raised by my parents to have a philanthropic mindset. As I mentioned, our one-income family had financial challenges, as do most people—yet my parents were always very giving and set a good example for me. They taught me to be philanthropic in word and deed, regardless of financial circumstances.

After all, "helping" does not have to involve cash. Not everyone has money to spare, and throwing money at a problem is not always the best way to solve it. Instead, if you can pinpoint an item or service that would benefit someone in need, it might do more to help them in the long run. Teaching someone a skill to help them get back on their feet may be the biggest and most welcome gift ever.

---

45 Merriam-Webster Dictionary, (n.d.). *Merriam-Webster Dictionary.* Definition of "Philanthropy." https://www.merriam-webster.com/dictionary/philanthropy.

Mask Up; Take Care of Yourself so You Can Take Care of Others!

Remember what they say on airplanes—secure your own oxygen mask before attempting to aid others. This will put you way ahead of the game when it comes to providing help and support.

It's impossible to see to others while you are struggling to breathe—and the same applies (in a metaphorical way) on a philanthropic level. It is not greedy to ensure you have your basic needs met before you reach out to help others. Otherwise, you're merely trading places with them, which puts both of you in a bad situation. Rather than solving someone else's problem, you aggravate your own.

Don't sacrifice yourself, despite how noble it may sound. You cannot give financially if you don't have a pot to you-know-what in, and you can't focus your energies on others if life is sapping your energy completely.

Care First

It's easy to care for someone's plight when it's also your own. It's harder to put yourself in someone else's shoes.

The key to providing targeted help to those in need is to care about them and their struggles on a deep, personal level. But how do you learn to care? How do you build compassion?

The first step is to see others as human beings, people just like you. Not as "needy people" or do-good cases you can take on and try to fix, but fundamentally as other human beings, no different from you except for their circumstances.

When clients walk into my nonprofit dental clinic, I take time to talk with them. Sure, it's difficult to have a meaningful conversation when they've got buzzing tools inside their mouths, but communicating is the best way to humanize each other and make it easier to relate to one another. It helps me to see them as *people* instead of *clients*.

One way I connect with people, especially when they are captive audiences in my dental chair, is to help them relax by telling jokes. Here's one of my favorites:

Three Jewish mothers are sitting on a bench, arguing over whose son loves her the most. The first one says, "You know, my son sends me flowers every Shabbos."

"You call that love?" scoffs the second mother. "My son calls me every day!"

"That's nothing," says the third woman. "My son is in therapy five days a week. And the whole time, he only talks about me!"

Finding a way to connect with those in need can often do just as much good as any other act of kindness. Always try to establish a connection.

ALL WORK AND NO PLAY

The word "play" calls to mind children rushing about, laughing and screeching, or racing and tumbling. Or perhaps you imagine sullen teens deep into their video games, with the occasional grunt of triumph as they progress a level.

Excuse me while I turn to the *Merriam-Webster Dictionary* as it weighs in on *play*: "to play in sport or recreation, frolic."[46]

In other words, the concept of play can be applied to almost anything that isn't work or some other specific responsibility—unless, of course, your work is that fortunate instance of being

---

46   Merriam-Webster Dictionary (n.d.). *Merriam-Webster Dictionary*. Definition of "Play." https://www.merriam-webster.com/dictionary/play.

paid to do what you love most, in which case you never have to "work" a day in your life.

There are two kinds of play—active and passive. Active play is something that, as the phrase suggests, gets and keeps you engaged on a physical or mental level, such as sports or video games. Inactive play includes passive activities such as watching television or listening to music. A balanced, happy life includes both.

When you've had a physically or mentally draining day, inactive play gives you a chance to rest and recover so you can start fresh tomorrow. When your day has been sluggish, with not much going on, active play can be a pick-me-up that gives you the spark you've been lacking.

Depending on the play you engage in, these activities can also count toward your daily exercise. Way to multitask!

We often encourage kids to enjoy themselves, usually while reminding them that they won't be able to do that as much when they're older. On some level, that is correct—as an adult, you bear more responsibilities. But playtime is just as important for adults as a way of rewarding mind, body, and spirit. In the absence of a schoolteacher telling us it's time for recess, we have to learn to set aside adult playtime for ourselves.

In his book *Die with Zero*, Bill Perkins shares an interesting theory: that the business of life is the acquisition of memories.[47] That thought has stuck with me.

---

47   Perkins, Bill (2020). *Die with Zero*. Mariner Books.

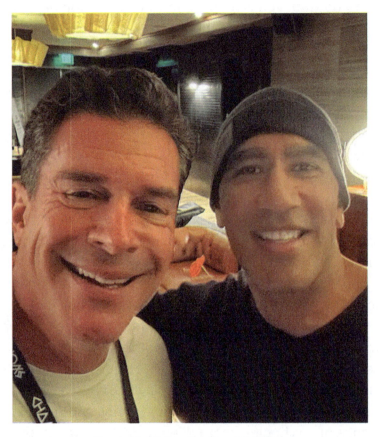

Figure 16: Dr. J and author Bill Perkins

In younger years, when income is usually minimal, saving money is a challenge and often goes on the back burner. As you go on in life and become more accomplished—with your income increasing commensurately—it's easier to put money away. But consider this: is it always of the utmost importance to try to save for a rainy day when you're young? What about using some of your limited funds while you're young to travel, and have adventures, and do the things you won't be able to do as much once you get married, start raising a family, and clock in at a full-time job?

My wife and I are in the process of examining our resources and deciding how best to use them for building our own memories, including gifting resources to our kids while we're still around to see the benefits. Perkins says the best time to gift people is when they are between the ages of twenty-five and forty—the time your children are most in need of supplementary resources, such as a deposit on a home. If you wait until you die, perhaps in your eighties, your children will be about in their fifties or sixties and likely will not need as much help as when they were starting out in life and career.

Don't wait until you're six feet under to enjoy, in real time, the memories and bonds you can build with others.

Why is play important? Much like other forms of relaxation, it helps both body and brain de-stress by removing them from the grind of the usual activities and environments that put pressure on them.

Think about a time when you spent an entire week doing nothing but working or studying. Exhausting, am I right? Sometimes you have no choice but to put in extra time and effort toward something, but there's no need to make constant productivity a habit. All you'll get is burnout, and then you're of no use to yourself or others. Where's that airplane oxygen mask when you need it?

Pushing too hard for too long leads to burnout. Burnout typically comes from doing things you don't enjoy doing. Maybe you don't enjoy them physically or you don't feel appropriately compensated. Whatever the case, this kind of activity saps your motivation and passion, silences innovation and creativity, and can, in some cases, lead to a lower sense of self-esteem through the misbegotten belief that you are, in some way, lazy or incapable.

Is it burnout? Is it depression? Sometimes it is both.

When you feel burned out by your job, the first thing to do is take a break. Once you have some breathing space, ask yourself whether you would enjoy the work more if it paid better. If yes, find a way to increase the value of what you charge or to present your value in a juicier way as you ask for a raise. If no, begin the process of researching a way to transition into another venture or activity, either temporarily or permanently.

I find that in dentistry, whenever I start to feel burnout, I put more time into Homeless Not Toothless, my nonprofit.

I love dentistry—making a difference for others, getting people out of pain, and giving people a smile that inspires and thrills them. But, as in any profession, there are things I don't like. In dentistry, that involves dealing with insurance companies and patient financial matters. Even people who love their work can be prone to burnout, and often it has to do with exhaustion and impatience with the finances of the business.

The mistake many people make, especially caregivers, is neglecting to schedule time for themselves, either as individuals or together. Even if you don't have children, it's important to set boundaries that insist on "time off" for yourself, to be with friends, or to enjoy your family. In a society that is so focused on productivity—of more, faster, better, higher—it is vital to step back now and again to reboot your body and mind.

You don't need to be entirely alone in a room or submerged in a sensory deprivation tank for it to count as "me time." Maybe utter solitude is exactly what you need sometimes, but you can also have quality "me time" simply by doing an activity you crave and enjoy. Reading a new book by a favorite author. Catching up on cat memes. What makes it "me time" is doing something you like, with or without company, with no external expectations.

You'll also want to incorporate "we time," to enjoy spending nonwork time with others.

Some people dance it off. Jog it off. Active play can be joyous and explosive, but sometimes, the perfect way to recharge those mental and physical batteries is by settling in with someone you enjoy spending time with and doing, perhaps, a whole lotta nothing. Talking, laughing, zoning out, or ... a whole lotta nothing. Heavenly. There's no right or wrong way to relax with the people you care about.

I incorporate play into my week, every week, without fail. I want to know that when I leave this world, I contributed to society, and to my family, and that I enjoyed the ride.

Too many people wait until it's too late to play. They risk missing out on it altogether.

Finding the Right Balance for YOU

The world around us has become so focused on doing and having more that it's difficult not to feel guilty when you want or need a break. It's gotten so bad that there are stories of people who work from their hospital beds because of the pressures of our work culture. But finding a work-life balance is not just a lovely idea—it's vital for your physical and mental health.

No one can set boundaries for you, and no one can enforce them on your behalf. If you don't set and maintain your own limits between personal and professional, you won't be able to function fully in either realm. Eventually, stress and fatigue will win and take you down with them.

My frequent exhaustion has a lot to do with running on all cylinders and rarely taking a break. It also has a lot to do with the numerous spine surgeries that have given me constant pain and muscle restraints since 2010. I literally have not had a day without pain for the past fourteen years, which is draining, to say the least, in every way.

I have found that my body responds very well to power naps, whereas my wife cannot nap without it ruining her sleep later—naps actually drain her. I once told my acupuncturist, Diane Black, how upset I was that I needed to nap, and she replied, "Wow, aren't you lucky? You can refuel yourself in fifteen minutes!" With that, I had a new paradigm through which to look at life; suddenly, my daily exhaustion had a solution.

I was stunned. I had been blind to the blessing. I couldn't see this "gift" for what it was until someone else pointed it out. DaVinci, Aristotle, Winston Churchill, Albert Einstein—even Kanye West—were all famous fans of the power nap. I now plan on having one most days, and through it, I get the benefit of being refueled.

Here are some hacks for better sleep:

- Must be tracked, just like all other important areas of your life; personally, I use the Oura Ring.
- The temperature of the room when sleeping is ideally between 60 and 67 degrees.
- Eat most or all of your food when it is light outside, and do not eat anything starting three to five hours prior to bedtime.
- Avoid alcohol and caffeine at least three hours prior to bedtime.
- Avoid technology (screens) for at least two hours before bedtime.
- Mollie Eastman has an awesome podcast on sleep called *Sleep Is a Skill*.[48]

What are some ways in which you enjoy taking a break, even if others rib you for it as being lazy or strange?

---

48 Eastman, Mollie (n.d.). *Sleep Is a Skill*. "Sleep Is a Skill." https://www.sleepisaskill.com/about.

Start Each Day Right

Hal Elrod's book *The Miracle Morning* focuses on how to begin each and every day with calm, clarity, and confidence.[49] He believes in the power of your inner world and the impact it has on your outer world, which lines up nicely with the connections among the **Essential Pillars**.

Elrod teaches the six Life SAVERS: Silence, Affirmations, Visualization, Exercise, Reading, and Scribing.[50] Each requires as little as ten minutes a day, and you can customize the routine to work with your lifestyle and goals.

1. **Silence.** Once you leave your bed and start your day, finding true quiet in which to collect yourself is difficult. Elrod recommends taking advantage of that moment of silence first thing in the morning and mixing in elements of prayer, meditation, reflection, gratitude, and breath control.

2. **Affirmations**. Self-talk and subconscious programming can wreak havoc with our mindset, performance, and results. Take stock of what runs through your head to help manage and mold the attitude you wish to have for the rest of the day.

3. **Visualization.** Some call this "manifestation." If you've read *The Secret* by Rhonda Byrne, you'll understand this task well. It involves building a mental visual of the kinds of progress and success you wish to experience in the real world, which—in itself—brings you closer to it.

---

49 Elrod, Hal (2023). *The Miracle Morning*. BenBella Book.
50 Elrod, Hal (n.d.). *The Miracle Morning*. "SAVERS". https://miraclemorning.com/episode-25-the-6-life-savers-for-a-miracle-morning/.

4. **Exercise.** You cannot hear this enough: getting your body moving boosts your energy, health, and concentration.

5. **Reading.** This keeps your mind healthy the same way food keeps your body healthy. Feed your mind, feed your body.

6. **Scribing.** Elsewhere, people generally refer to this as "journaling." Writing down your thoughts and feelings to review later is a great way to declutter and organize your mind. Your brain is for having ideas, not holding ideas. You must get your thoughts out of your head as quickly as possible—write them down so that they are memorialized, therefore freeing up your brain to have new ideas.

Elrod's advice has become a staple of my own daily routine. Now, I'm in bed by 10:00 p.m.—I'll even turn off a TV show midway to honor my bedtime.

I sleep with a face mask and earplugs so I can stay in a deep sleep, uninterrupted by light or noise. As I describe in my Time Blocking chart, I awaken at 5:30 a.m. most days—6:00 a.m. if I'm "sleeping in"—and begin my morning routine. Because my body has taken a beating over the years, I soak in a hot tub for at least forty-five minutes to limber up. I have a cup of coffee and my laptop with me in the Jacuzzi, where I go through my email and respond only to those that will take a few seconds to reply to; the rest can wait for later. I also review my banking to ensure my financial commitments are on firm ground for that day and week.

Next, it's off to the gym for cardio and weights. I finish in the sauna for twenty minutes to sweat it all out and meditate.

After this two-hour ritual, I feel accomplished, alert, and ready for the day.

There are endless techniques for transforming and even ending your challenges with sleeping, and you've probably heard of many of them. Here are a few that come to mind, although not everything on my list is right for yours:

- Get therapy
- Drink green tea
- Meditate
- Take transformational courses
- Visit Tibet, hang with monks
- Get your meridians balanced
- Consult an astrologer and get your palm read
- Find religion
- Go vegetarian
- Take cold showers
- Write affirmations
- Make a vision board

And there's a plethora of other ways. In the end, while they all have the possibility to work, it ultimately comes down to finding the path best suited for you and declaring that you'll stay on that path until you reach the goal or level of freedom you seek.

An Attitude of Gratitude

Part of my daily morning routine is the act of gratitude, something that did not always come naturally to me. Over time, though, I have been able to use the act of gratitude to focus on what I can be doing with my time on Earth instead of giving in to frustration. The actions I take include everything from helping others via philanthropic causes and ensuring my family has a legacy, to taking courses and attending seminars to expand my leadership abilities. It was through my concentration on gratitude that I was able to start Homeless Not Toothless.

Trip to Hungary

When I learned through DNA matching that I was 50 percent Hungarian, I decided to visit the home of my ancestors. One of the amazing results of my trip to Hungary and Austria for my fiftieth birthday was an adventure to Salzburg, where my father served in the Army during the Korean War.

Usually a quiet man, my dad always spoke about his years in Europe with tremendous admiration and joy. When Briar and I visited the Army base where he'd been stationed, I was taking photos from the street when an Austrian military policeman approached. He asked what I was doing, to which I replied I wanted to show my dad the places he had loved decades ago.

The MP called his commander, who shortly thereafter showed up in his vehicle.

"Would you please tell your father we thank him for his service? We are grateful for all America has done to support us," he said. "Would you like a tour of the base?"

A veteran myself, I am still moved by the gratitude of others when they acknowledge what the U.S. military has done for them. Even as I write about this many years later, a thrill runs through my veins. This was one of the highlights of my life—the opportunity to visit a place my father held so dear to his heart, and to be welcomed there so warmly. My gratitude is boundless.

Embracing the concept of gratitude is simple in theory, but a bear to put into practice—let alone making it a habit. It's not always easy to be grateful for everything that happens in our lives, but there are many types of gratitude that we can use to help us out.

But first—why is gratitude so important?

Think about it. When you do something for someone and receive heartfelt thanks for your effort, how does that make you feel? Warm and fuzzy, yes? Wrapped in a cocoon of positive energy? It revs up a lovely cycle of giving and receiving and generates love and hope.

Now that we know why gratitude is important, let's explore the four basic types of gratitude—none of them better or worse than the others. All are important in creating a habit of gratitude and funneling goodwill into your storage of karma:

- **Anticipatory:** when you're thankful for something that hasn't yet happened.
- **Retrospective:** when you're thankful for something that happened in the past.
- **Global:** when you're thankful for everything in your life that lends it meaning and dimension.
- **Active:** when you're thankful for something right now, in the very moment it is happening.

"Okay," you say. "I'm sold on gratitude. When should I practice it?"

Every single day.

Gratitude is not a one-time thing. It's like eating to stay healthy: you need to repeat it consistently, for your benefit and for the benefit of the people around you. I strongly recommend that part of your daily routine—perhaps upon waking or right before going to sleep—includes a moment of gratitude.

You can express gratitude in many simple ways, from saying "thank you" to your significant other for making breakfast to journaling or praying or giving back—that's right, philanthropy is a form of gratitude. How? You're taking your extra resources and ensuring they don't go to waste. It shows you understand the value of things, even if they are things that you don't personally need.

The End of Mrs. Killjoy

We have discussed mentors and gratitude. I'd like to tie those two together by sharing two very different legacies from two of my high school teachers. You've already heard how one of them, the English teacher Mrs. Killjoy, cut me down, but allow me to elaborate a bit.

At the time, I was neither an athlete nor a nerd—just someone who blended in and went along largely unnoticed. I had not yet made my mark or even knew where I might make one.

Once I realized that becoming a doctor might be my way forward, I began studying harder and participating more in class. That's why I raised my hand when Mrs. Killjoy had each of us read a paragraph aloud from a book and answer questions about the content.

The answer I gave was a literal translation of the passage, but the teacher thought the author was being facetious and that I hadn't picked up on the nuance. For that sin, she announced to the class, "Grossman, you will never amount to anything."

Between her assessment of my future and my classmates laughing, I felt more than embarrassed. I felt destroyed. Maybe she was right—that I would never become a doctor or anything of note. That I didn't have the right.

A few weeks later, my social studies teacher pulled me aside. We had received our first test back. I'd gotten an eighty-eight, which I was pretty happy with—until the teacher dismissed the class early, saying, "Everyone but Jay is free to go. Jay, come to my office."

As my social studies teacher lit his pipe in his tiny office (yes, teachers were allowed to smoke in school in the 1970s), he said, "I was thinking about failing you on this test," to which I protested, "But I didn't cheat!"

"I didn't say you did," he said. "But I know you didn't study, either."

The blood drained from my face. I'd shown my hand, and he was right. I hadn't studied.

All I could think to say was, "How did you know?"

He turned his grade book toward me and said, "Find your name."

I did, and I noticed two marks next to it. Both were eighty-eight. He explained that the first grade was the one he anticipated the student would get based on classroom participation. So, clearly, he thought I had walked into the class with an eighty-eight already in my pocket—which is why he (accurately) believed I hadn't studied, or I would have surpassed his baseline expectation.

Now, *this* was a real teacher!

He then asked what I wanted to do with my life. I told him I was thinking of becoming a dentist.

"Do you think an eighty-eight is a sufficient grade to get you into a good medical program?" he asked.

This was a mic-drop moment for me, as I'd never asked myself that question. It hadn't occurred to me.

With that, my social studies teacher tossed me the Yellow Pages—a thick book containing contact information for area businesses, from back in the days before the internet—and said, "Let's call a local dentist and ask."

I found a full-page ad for the pediatric dentist Dr. Charles Pillar—yup, "Pillar" was his name, as if anticipating this book decades later—and called the number.

A woman named Margie answered the phone. I introduced myself as a high school student down the street from their office and explained that my teacher wanted a moment of the doctor's time. I handed the phone to my teacher, and they engaged in a short conversation that went something like this:

"Dr. Pillar? My name is Mr. Boss, and I have what is possibly our school valedictorian standing in front of me. He wants to become a dentist, and we have a new externship program where the students leave campus for half a day each week. I wanted to ask if you were willing to take him on, if you'd have the ability to mentor him and show him what dentistry is all about. Inspire him. Would you consider helping?"

I'd never heard of this program. After the call, I asked my teacher how long this wonderful, innovative program had been around. He looked at his watch and said, "It started five minutes ago."

In a matter of moments, my world had righted itself. Despite my English teacher's harsh opinion of me, I also had a teacher who thought I had the potential to be a valedictorian. His comments empowered me and put me on the path I am on now.

That externship program changed my life. I fell in love with the profession of dentistry and, lo and behold, took all of my studies more seriously. This type of teaching, caring, and dedication—as opposed to Mrs. Killjoy's scorched-earth policy—so inspired me that I have taught and lectured since 1992 with the express hope of likewise empowering, inspiring, and motivating others. I want to help them take business seriously; be more accepting, understanding, and forgiving; and make the world a better place overall, just as Mr. Boss had done for me. That is also why I started my nonprofit so that I can give back.

Giving back is the most worthwhile endeavor I have found—but to do it, first, you need to make enough money so that your bills are taken care of and you're not worried about the mortgage. Put your own oxygen mask on first if you intend to be philanthropic.

I was thrilled when I first stepped into the dental office of Dr. Charlie Pillar in Plainview, New York, as a fifteen-year-old high school student. I sat chairside and was able to assist with small things, such as suctioning and general organization.

Charlie launched my motivation to continue doing better in my studies. He showed me the benefit dentistry provides to his patients and how running a successful office allows you to have an extraordinary life. He also talked about his education at the NYU College of Dentistry, which of course became my focused goal, and the only dental school to which I wanted to apply. I'm still in touch with him and still grateful for that externship, as it helped me choose a field that, decades later, I still love. In fact, one of the reasons I have had thousands of students come through my office was to pay it forward, as Dr. Charlie did for me.

Just as empowering, I took my failure in tenth-grade English, which haunted me, and turned it around. It seems only fair that I have made the journey from being told that my interpretation of a book was incorrect to now, when—in my work as an expert witness—I am asked for my opinion (my interpretation, if you will) of what I am reading. And with more than a thousand cases under my belt, clearly, lawyers see value in my interpretation.

My interpretation. Not Mrs. Killjoy's.

Gratitude heals your body by causing the release of healing hormones such as dopamine and serotonin. These hormones help you physically and emotionally, which improves your mood and makes it easier to adopt new, healthy habits.

HURDLES

In 2010, when I was forty-seven, I got into a head-on accident while I was driving to work at fifty miles per hour on the highway. The other guy was on the wrong side of the road, traveling north in the south-bound lane.

I woke up in an ambulance, somehow still alive. Both shoulders were dislocated and needed surgical repair, and the force of the impact caused my colon to herniate. I also had testicular damage and herniated cervical and lumbar discs, all requiring surgery.

I missed years of work as I struggled to recover. It wasn't just the bed rest; I also had a slew of surgeries over the years, including removing a mass from my tongue caused by pressure from the tube used to intubate me during one surgery, causing permanent numbness on the right-hand side of my tongue. I received artificial replacements in multiple parts of my spine, and these substitutes, while miraculous, will always limit my movements. All the surgeries resulted in a vast network of scar tissue that limits mobility and requires an hour in the morning soaking in hot water so I can ambulate.

Recently, I had lumbar nerves burned to reduce my back pain, and will probably have this procedure repeated yearly. I have also had a permanent nerve stimulator installed in my spine with battery packs that will need additional surgeries to replace as the battery fails. I'm not exactly plug-and-play.

As I write this book, fourteen years after the accident, I am still in daily pain and am probably not done with surgeries.

If you enjoyed my previous drawing of a marketing funnel, you're gonna love these photos:

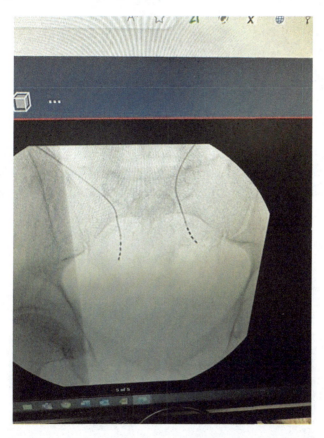

Figure 17: Spinal nerve stimulation probes that are constantly sending shocks to my spinal cord

This is an image of the spinal nerve stimulator in my lumbar/pelvic region, controlled by a phone app. This helps control my bladder, which was affected by the hardware in my lumbar spine. I have a medical card to show the TSA because I light up their sensors when I fly.

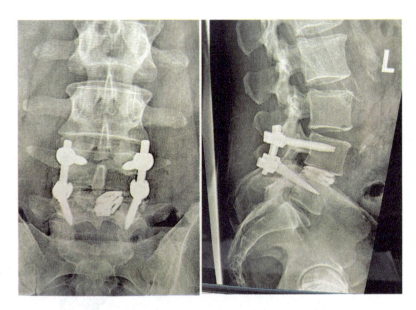

Figures 18: Lumbar fixation due to car accident

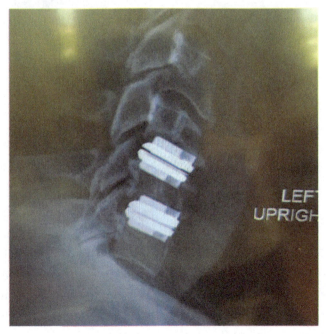

Figure 19: Cervical disk replacement due to car accident

After the accident, it became even more important for Briar and me to work consistently on our communication. That my life could have ended on that highway was another wake-up call, reminding me how much I loved my wife and how much work I had yet to do on my Personal pillar. If I did not give daily gratitude for having lived through a head-on collision on the highway, I would be in a deep, dark hole.

I was not out of the woods yet. After all those procedures, we'd all somehow still missed that a concussion had begun to affect my memory—and had led to some dark thoughts.

I had just gotten a lift home from one of my many medical appointments a few months post-accident when Briar asked, "Where's the milk?"

"Probably in the fridge," I replied.

I didn't understand her frustration until she explained that we'd had a phone conversation only fifteen minutes prior in which she'd asked me to pick up a container on my way home. I didn't remember the contents of the conversation—or that we'd even had one.

The memory struggles continued to confuse me, to the point where I questioned whether I'd actually survived the crash and instead was stuck in some kind of afterlife.

There was a day shortly after the accident when I caught myself looking out my office window and thinking, "I should jump." It wasn't even about trying to hurt myself. My thoughts at the time were dark and jumbled, and somehow, I thought that jumping would either prove or disprove my endless-loop theory about how maybe I had died in the crash after all. Since nothing made sense to me at that time, this thought seemed as reasonable as any other.

Thankfully, I was strong enough to fight against that idea. Instead, I called a psychiatrist who had an office in the same building.

"Hi, Stephen, it's Jay from downstairs. I'm thinking about jumping out the window. Can you give me a call back?"

As I write this, I can't imagine what a psychiatrist would think when a new patient calls, saying they are about to jump out a window! As you can imagine, Dr. Stephen Poulter called me right back and had me come to his office immediately.

After hearing what was going on with me, he explained that there was likely a brain swelling causing some memory loss from a lack of enough oxygen squeezing through. He added that it might also explain my thundercloud thoughts.

I am forever grateful to Dr. Poulter for literally saving my life that day.

I signed up for therapy. On a whim, I asked my father one time if he'd like to join me for a therapy session, as he was in the office for a dental cleaning, and we had a lunch date I had forgotten when I scheduled the appointment. I doubted he'd be up for it.

To my surprise, he agreed.

I was in for another surprise. During the session, the therapist asked my dad what it was like to raise me, and the answer was unexpected, to say the least—given that he wasn't the most overtly affectionate person.

"It was the best time of my life," my dad said.

Then, the therapist asked what my father did for a living, and his answer was so surprising, I was afraid I'd turn into Linda Blair in *The Exorcist*, my head spinning round and round.

"Oh, I was really fortunate," said my dad. "I had the best job in the world. I made enough to pay the bills, and that allowed me to be home every day to give my son a bath before dinner."

It wasn't until then that I realized why my father had never sought out a different, higher-paying job. He'd made an active choice to put quality time with his family ahead of making money. I also began to see and appreciate the choices and sacrifices my parents made, including my stay-at-home mom managing—while raising my sister and me—to earn her master's degree.

"Dad, why didn't you ever tell me this before?" I sputtered.

"You were on your own path," he said. "I had faith you'd be able to figure things out for yourself."

My father passed away a few months later from leukemia.

Sometimes, we don't realize something is a blessing in disguise until much later. That's how I feel now about my car accident. Without it leading me to therapy, I might never have learned the depths to which my father loved and cared for his family and his viewpoint on what mattered most before he died.

What difficulty have you come to realize was a blessing in disguise?

PERSONAL EXERCISE 1:
Get on Track[51]

Just as you can track your finances, you can track elements of your Personal pillar. Rate yourself on a scale of zero to ten.

Track your workout routine. How many days do you plan to commit to exercise, and how many days do you fulfill that promise? I suggest exercising a minimum of three times per week and pushing yourself up to five

---

51 Dr. Jay Grossman, (n.d.). #8. *Essential Pillars* Personal Exercise 1, Average Life Happiness Index. www.drjaydds.com.

times a week. Also, rate yourself on the frequency and intensity of exercise.

Track your self-help, growth, and development. What is your commitment to growing yourself? Whether it's taking a seminar or reading a book, track it!

Track your meditation practice. Devote at least ten minutes a day to freeing your mind, either through guided imagery or free-association. The brain has a very hard time distinguishing between reality and fantasy, which is why dreams seem so real. Setting your parameters for the day and having positive affirmations gets your brain to believe it's real, which is a great way to get on track toward accomplishing your goals.

Track your nutrition: are you eating healthily? Making smart food choices? You can track how many ounces of water you've consumed, how many servings of vegetables and fruits you've eaten, and roughly how many ounces of protein you're getting per day. Are you at your ideal weight? You can rate yourself on metrics of your own devising—but rate yourself on a numbered scale and without editorializing via unhelpful comments, like: "I ate like a pig today!"

Where do you stand on spirituality? If it is part of your routine, track it. Are you clear about your purpose in life? Are you on track for your vision? Are you happy? Assign it a number and see how and whether that changes over time.

You can add or delete to this list as it suits you. Some people have "dance" on their exercise list in a section on hobbies. Dancing is not on my scorecard because my surgeries prevent me from partaking—but, let's face it, dancing was never my forte. You wouldn't have wanted to see me tango, even in the best of times. Instead, I actually track the amount of pain I am in, as I am committed to getting *out* of pain. Today, on my list, I have a score of three out of ten for painlessness, meaning that I have a long way to go to get to a pain-free ten.

By looking at my Personal pillar scorecard, I can clearly see what still needs work. I have included time spent in dollar-productive activities, love for my work, and how much I'm feeding my love of adventure, vacation, and travel. You can add things that excite you in life, and how much time you carve out to chill and unwind.

FOURTEEN CHILDREN

Several times a day, patients ask me about the many photos of my many children on the walls of my office.

"Yes," I say with pride, "I had fourteen kids with ten women in a twelve-year period, and I only learned about six of the children in 2019 and five more in 2024. It turns out that they were all born during the first five years of my marriage to Briar."

My patients are usually stunned. "Um, what does your wife think about that?" they ask.

"When I told her, she said it was the best day of her life."

Some of them tell me I must have a very open and liberal wife. Others say she probably had affairs herself, and this news lets her off the hook.

But a few of them get it right: "Were you by any chance a sperm donor?"

I always get a kick out of this. So does my wife (although the joke is getting old for her).

Together, Briar and I have three amazing biological children—Sydney, Eric, and Ari. But before we got married and started our family, back when I was twenty-one and still in dental school—living, like most struggling students, on bad coffee and cheap ramen noodles—I learned that being a sperm donor meant helping people who could not have children *and* receiving a paycheck as part of the deal. I was all for it.

I donated many times and went about my life—graduating, marrying, joining the Navy, and building my practices. Donor # C380 was my sperm donor number. Along the way, I forgot all about those long-ago sperm donations.

Until the DNA-matching website 23andMe started to gain traction.

23andMe intrigued me. I wanted to know more about my heritage. I paid for a kit and spat into a cup. My results came back showing that my heritage was 99 percent Russian, Hungarian, and Jewish, which wasn't exactly surprising but still a fun fact. I absorbed the news and didn't give the process much thought.

When I found out about these newly found children through 23andMe, it meant more love and more opportunities to be in relationships.

In 2018, I received a call from my sister-in-law Laura, who had quite the shock in store for me: one of the offspring from my sperm donations had reached out to her to contact me.

It seems Will had known since the age of ten that he had a sperm-donor dad out there somewhere, but he didn't pursue it until the father who raised him died so as not to upset him. Will lives in Missouri, has a wife and two adorable little girls, and is a successful architect who builds stadiums. In his efforts to contact me, he somehow found out that his sister-in-law got a dog from a breeder who is friends with the breeder Laura (my sister-in-law) used when she got her own puppy. Small world! He found this out by doing a Facebook search for me, as I only had my name and occupation listed on 23andMe with no other contact information.

Once Will tracked down Laura, he asked whether she knew if I had donated sperm in my youth. "Sounds like something he'd do," she said. I'm still not sure what Laura meant by that, but I'm going to assume it's complimentary.

After Laura gave me the stunning news, I logged back into 23andMe and found an avalanche of email notifications. Will wasn't my only progeny out there. My daughter-in-law, Brit, was with me at the time, and she immediately poured me a triple scotch. (When the scotch is from my liquor cabinet, she is very generous with the pour.)

"What are you going to do?" she asked.

"Call Briar," I said.

I was nervous about how my wife would react, but I needn't have been.

"I was wondering when they were going to show up," she said.

It turned out Briar thought it was really cool that I'd been able to help others have families of their own. She has since pointed out that our daughter, Sydney, and her wife, Brit, have given us three grandchildren with the help of a sperm donor. She cannot imagine a bigger gift than bringing life into the world for others.

And, yes, there were others. Apparently, I have given this gift to at least six families—and who knows if there are more!

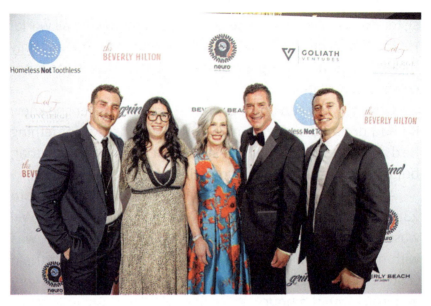

Figure 20: My immediate family: Ari, Sydney, wife Briar, Dr. J, and Eric

And here are nine of the fourteen children of mine (that I know of), from oldest to youngest. (As this book was being published, I learned about five more children and did not know them well enough, nor have their permission to write about them yet.):

LIZ (No. 1 of 9)

My oldest child is an actress in New York. Her father remarried when she was eighteen and, unfortunately, did not continue to pursue a relationship with Liz. Her mom died of pancreatic cancer after surviving Stage 4 inflammatory breast cancer. After DNA testing, Liz learned that she had the BRCA2 gene, a mutation that increases the odds of developing breast, ovarian, and pancreatic cancer.

After seeing what her mother had gone through, Liz coura-geously chose to have a prophylactic double mastectomy. She shared this with me on our first phone call, and we both got teary—me with pride in my newfound daughter for making such a bold, life-saving move and her because she had not expected such a positive response from the biological dad she had never met. I shared with her that my wife had had to make the same choice fifteen years prior, as my wife too is BRCA positive; fortunately, we caught her cancer at Stage 1. We are big fans of choosing life over aesthetics.

"Let me see if I have this right," said Liz. "You are my biological father, without any known medical issues, and you are willing to have a relationship with me? And your wife knows that you were a sperm donor and is also excited about welcoming me into the family?"

"That sounds about right, yes," I said.

"I was an orphan just minutes ago and now I have bio-parents and siblings? And you understand the BRCA mutation and support my medical decision?"

"Right again."

"Did I just hit the lottery?"

"I think we both did," I said, wiping away tears.

JORDAN (No. 2 of 9)

My second daughter is in a throuple relationship. She is married to James, and they both have Sara in their lives—hence, they are a throuple. I had already read Esther Perel's *Mating in Captivity*, which opened me up to the concept that sex, intimacy, and long-term relationships don't always follow pre-conceived notions. Briar and I had no issues with their arrangement, and that seemed to soften things immediately.

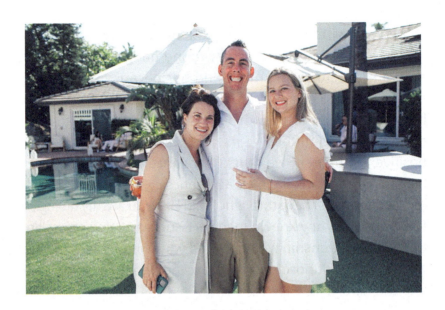

Figure 21: Jordan, James, Sara

The three of them live in Arizona and visit L.A. often, as Sara's parents live here. She has a brother who is also a donor child from another donor.

Jordan's girlfriend was diagnosed with leukemia in 2022, and I've been privileged to recommend doctors for her treatments and see them frequently when they are in L.A., which is several times a year. The outpouring of support for Sara by all of my children has been nothing short of extraordinary, and when the doctors declared Sara "cured," there were tears of joy all around. We threw a surprise party to celebrate when seven of the nine children were able to be in town.

MAX (No. 3 of 9)

My oldest son knew early on that he was a donor baby, as he was the son of two mothers. He went through most of his childhood without telling other kids about his family situation, as both of his mothers worked at schools in conservative institutions, and he didn't want to put their jobs at risk. Their employment contracts had a clause that said if they were gay, they could lose their jobs, so Max had the burden of keeping this secret, even from his close friends.

Max was the last of the newfound children to contact me and was thrilled to learn he had eight siblings; he invited the whole crew of us to his wedding to see Laura and him exchange vows. It was the first time all nine of my kids were in one place at the same time. I keep copies of a photo of the nine of them plastered everywhere—in an album, on my phone, framed on my desk—wherever I can, so I can see it regularly. (As of 2024, there are now fourteen children).

Max and Laura are both special education teachers on Long Island. In 2023, they welcomed Lucas, my ninth grandchild, into the world.

HILARY (No. 4 of 9)

Hilary has the strongest New York accent! She grew up from the age of fourteen with a single mom after her dad's abusive behavior led to divorce. She wasn't aware that there was a sperm donor in the picture until later, but once we spoke, when she was thirty, she was relieved to find me mentally healthy, as she had feared her father's violent nature would be passed down to her in a genetic soup.

Hilary—who attended SUNY Albany, where I did two years of undergraduate study—lives in upstate New York, works in real estate insurance, and has also been involved in philanthropy for a long time. Despite her misgivings about relationships—based on what she had seen growing up—Hilary was able to form a solid bond with Andrew. He had his own demons to deal with, yet the two of them have worked it through in a healthy, successful way. It is a gift for me to see these two building a beautiful life together. I have, on several occasions, spent the night at their place, and I see them every time I'm in New York.

WILL (No. 5 of 9)

Will, from Missouri, looks more like me than any of my burgeoning brood, including the two boys I had with my wife. At first, that was scary. Now, I think it's super cool!

Will's parents needed a donor because the father was sterile from prior radiation treatments. Will, like Hilary, was happy to see what kind of genetics his birthright was: at the time I spoke to him in 2018, I was fifty-five, didn't take any meds, and still had all my hair. My surgeries and attendant health problems all stemmed from the one car accident, so genetics was not a concern.

Even more amazing, my favorite uncle was named Will, and if Briar and I had had another son, we would have named him the same!

The first time we met, I threw Will, his wife, Monica, and their two daughters, Brielle and Keely, in the deep end: I invited them to my fifty-fifth birthday party, where a hundred friends and family got to meet them all at once.

Below is my sixtieth birthday party, with seven out of my fourteen kids in attendance!

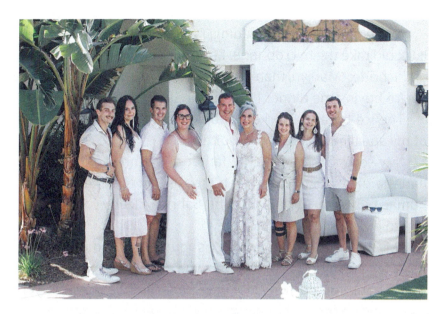

Figure 22: Dr. J's sixtieth birthday with seven of his fourteen children and wife Briar

SABRINA (No. 6 of 9)

Sabrina, my only Canadian daughter, has a fascinating story. Ten years ago, her father was dying of kidney disease. To save him, she secretly took a DNA test to see if she would be a match for a kidney transplant. That's how she learned he wasn't her biological parent—but she never told her parents about her knowledge so as not to upset them. She went on believing she was adopted until the day her father blurted out the whole truth.

Sabrina's mom, Marilyn, wasn't overly fond of the idea that Sabrina would be replacing her late father with a new one. So, when I was able to offer a toast at Sabrina's wedding to Mike—who also brought his two children, Jack and Carter, into the mix, along with Sabrina's daughter, Vienna—I was careful not to step on any toes.

In the middle of the wedding, I asked the bride and groom if I could take the microphone. My first toast was to the mother of the bride: "Marilyn, thank you for choosing me, but next time, you're buying me dinner first."

The ice-breaker worked. People laughed, and the anxiety of my speaking to the group softened.

"My second toast is to the father of the bride, who I never had the pleasure of meeting, but based on the extraordinary human being you turned out to be, Sabrina, clearly your parents did an excellent job raising you.

"My third toast is to all of you, as you have all come up to me, my wife, and my other six children who are here, to welcome us. And I thank you profusely for your generous welcome, as you have made a potentially awkward situation very comfortable."

I closed out with a toast to the bride and groom.

SYDNEY (No. 7 of 9)

My oldest daughter by my wife was my very first child—or so I thought until 23andMe set me straight.

Sydney and I share a remarkable father-daughter bond. We speak almost daily, see each other weekly, and she and her wife, Brit—my personal assistant and one of my wife's closest friends—have given me three beautiful grandchildren: Thea, Nathan, and Zoe. All three are from the same sperm donor, with the first two conceived with eggs from my daughter and the third with an egg from Brit. All of them were carried to term by Sydney. Thank goodness for modern medicine!

They all live a few minutes from us, so Briar and I get to be involved in their lives while taking care not to be overly intrusive.

Watching my baby girl become a woman and a mother has been one of the biggest joys of my life.

ERIC (No. 8 of 9)

My middle child, birthed by my wife, has had a challenging journey. Sadly, his girlfriend of eight years died from an overconsumption of alcohol, and it upended Eric's life. He took a needed year off to recalibrate and ultimately decided that law school was not for him. Instead, he is completing his master's degree in marriage and family therapy, having decided that his calling is to help others in likewise challenging circumstances. Today, he is in a healthy relationship with a wonderful young lady, and I am proud to watch him forging his own path.

ARI (No. 9 of 9)

My youngest child has had huge hurdles to overcome, including grappling with a seizure disorder that sent him to the hospital countless times with seizure-related incidents, including fractured teeth. I have to admire his incredible resilience in getting up every day and facing the world despite the chance that a seizure could have dire consequences. The way he has faced his challenges is inspirational and powerful.

We finally found the right doctor and the right medications. I wept when he made it through an entire year without any incidents.

Ari also turned around a childhood struggle with weight to become a physical fitness trainer—who is built like a brick you-know-what!

This photo was taken in 2019 at Max's wedding, where he invited ALL of his siblings. It was the first time all nine of my children met one another!

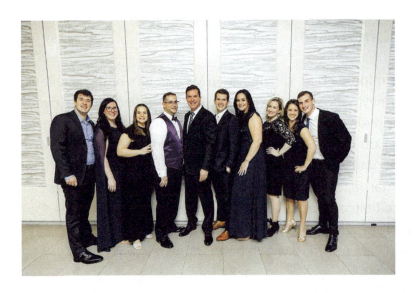

Figure 23: Dr. J's nine children (currently there are fourteen in total);
the first time they all met each other at Max's wedding in 2019

My three children with Briar call me Dad, and my other six rascals call me their "bio-dad." They all have my flat feet. They all have my dimples. They all have my charming personality—although Briar says they have it, and I don't. "Looks like it skipped a generation," she says.

Ha, she doesn't really say that! But she probably thinks it.

All my children have brought me a tremendous amount of joy, growth, and happiness—and, at times, appropriate worry and sorrow. I'm ridiculously proud of their journeys and who they've become, and I treasure the strong bond I have with them and the openness my bio-kids have with all their siblings, near and far.

I feel blessed, and I say that as an agnostic. I don't know how else to express it. Even though I didn't raise six of my bio-kids and didn't meet them until they were fully grown, I love them, and so does my wife, which truly speaks to how remarkable she is.

We have all celebrated weddings, birthdays, and anniversaries together. We have commemorated losses. We have become a "chosen family," in that we all choose each other exactly as we are.

It's a remarkable lovefest and one I wouldn't have been able to build and appreciate if I hadn't mastered my Personal pillar. Experiencing, appreciating, and holding close all the inevitable ups and downs of loving relationships is not second nature to most people. It takes work.

Even the heartaches are essential for personal growth and development. I encourage you to look back on your own trials and hardships with a new lens, with the perspective of the **Essential Pillars**, collectively and individually. It will help you rewire the pathways in your brain and turn negative experiences into opportunities for growth.

It's never too late.

Takeaways from the Personal Pillar

The Personal pillar deals with mind, body, and soul.

Rate yourself on each of the following individually, or give yourself an overall grade for this category on a scale of zero to ten. Factor in career, health, nutrition, exercise, recreation and vacations, the environment at home and at work, happiness, contentment, hobbies, risk tolerance, excitement, chill time, how you give back, and your gratitude.

Follow a ninety-minute rule of breaking off and taking a walk, or even just pacing around a bit, to stretch and distract mind and body for ten to fifteen minutes.

Develop a healthy "miracle morning" routine.

Where are you in terms of philanthropy? What are you doing to leave this planet better off than the way in which you found it?

Essential Pillars Personal Exercise 1, Average Life Happiness Index

as of	TODAY()

Happiness Index, Score 0 - low, 10 - hi	
	Diet / Water / Weight
	Exercise
	Dollar Productive Activities
	Love for Work
	Romance
	Relationship with Children
	Relationship with Parents/Siblings
	Relationship with Friends
	Horizontal Income
	Pain perceived by body
	Hobbies
	Adventure / Travel
	Risk & Excitement
	Chill Time
	Giving Back
	Future Planning
	Gratitude Thermometer
	Add your own criteria

#DIV/0!   Average Life Happiness Index

52   Dr. Jay Grossman, (n.d.). *Personal Pillar, Exercise #1. Average Life Happiness Index.* https://www.drjaydds.com/.

Conclusion

The **Essential Pillars**—Prosperity, People, and Personal—all exist and can function at a base level on their own. Their existence is not dependent on each other. However, to function at their best—and, therefore, for you to function at your best—all three need to be solid, strong, balanced structures.

Now that you have a good understanding of the **Essential Pillars**, you can use that knowledge to reinforce your business strategies and personal relationships, as well as your health and wellness. With a ton of books out there that drill into specific niches in each pillar, this book is designed to offer a global view, not a deep dive. Otherwise, the book would be thousands of pages long. My suggestion is that whenever you get to a specific area within a pillar where you're weak, explore it deeper with whatever resources you can find—be it a book I recommend in the Additional Reading section, a coach in that field, or from among the goodies a Google search unearths.

If you can master active handling of each pillar and all that the **Essential Pillars** encompass, you'll be rewarded with financial freedom, unbreakable relationships—and a long, fulfilling, healthy, and successful life.

Remember: If you struggle along the way, it's okay. You're human. Return to these pages anytime you need a refresher.

It is my hope that there are a few pearls in this book that make the time to read it worthwhile. Develop the discipline to consistently take the actions that will bring you the success you want and deserve. Being "normal" is often the aim of the unsuccessful; consider instead being "abnormal," doing more than others, and pushing beyond the norm.

I also welcome you to reach out to me directly. As an experienced lecturer and coach, I'm happy to answer any questions you might have. Here's how we can connect by email:

EssentialPillars@gmail.com

One final thought: I wrote this book after decades of procrastination because I still heard my English teacher's voice in my head: "Grossman, you will never amount to anything." Writing this book represents my personal breakthrough.

Also, though, it prompted me to think it through, and this is what I came up with: I've had plenty of success in life despite Mrs. Killjoy—or, perhaps, because of her. Every step along my path was to prove her wrong, and as a result, I'm grateful for that interaction with her. At the time, at fifteen years old, I was devastated by her comment, and I certainly don't condone her teaching style. Nevertheless, I'm happy and content with my path and where it's led, and that leaves me at peace with her and with the universe.

Acknowledgments

Writing a book takes a village, and I'd like to thank mine: my fourteen kids and my thirteen grandchildren. They all came into my life at various times and have been my true joy of being on this planet, and I thank them all for helping to give me a purpose.

Children (in chronological order): Liz, Dara, Alyssa, Jordan, Max, Hilary, Liz, Will, Sabrina, Sydney, Samantha, Eric, Victoria & Ari.

Grandchildren: Brielle, Keely, Vienna, Jack, Carter, Thea, Nathan, Zoe, Lucas, Ryhs, Chloe, Cooper & Cameron.

Thank you to my loving and courageous wife, Briar. Our journey together has been and continues to be one of never-ending love and surprise. You are the wind beneath my wings!

To my tremendous team of advisors, coaches, mentors, and friends: Igor Zey, Tony Principe, Larry Bernstein, Matt Johnson, Robert Chun, Elise Slifkin-McClure, Cameron Shayne, Zak Lee, Jen Herda, Dr. Charlie Pillar, Dr. Paul Lanza, Jeff Egol, Howard L. Kaplan, Jason Felson, Adam Rude, and Michael Levine. To my dental staff—many of you have been with me for twenty-five years; there are no words to thank you for your loyalty properly. Thank you all for the education of life and for your patience, coaching, training, and mentorship.

Also, a shout-out to my patient editors and proofreaders: Briar Grossman, Keidi Keating, Jami Bernard, Howard L. Kaplan, and Brett Levine.

My staff; without whom I would have had a miserable 30+ years in practice, they made going to work fun, enjoyable, and successful.

Special thanks to Kate L. Muffet, cover design.

About the Author

From the age of ten, Dr. Jay Grossman knew he wanted to be a dentist. He liked the idea of helping other people and saw firsthand from his own dentist, a family friend, that dentistry was the perfect career to make that happen. His undergraduate accomplishments and passion for dentistry led him to the New York University College of Dentistry, which accepted him at age nineteen before he completed his undergraduate degree.

At twenty-four, Dr. Grossman moved with his wife and newborn to Santa Monica, California, where he enlisted in the Navy—a dynamic venue that afforded him a plethora of experiences. After completing a tour of duty as a lieutenant in the Navy Dental Corps and receiving a National Defense Service Medal, he was profiled in major magazines as the new poster boy for recruitment, thanks to his innovative nonprofit, Homeless Not Toothless. He has received letters of commendation from President Obama, the Secretary of the Navy, and numerous members of Congress for his nonprofit. He started his own practice in 1991 in Brentwood, California, where he has been practicing ever since, with more than 15,000 loyal patients over the years, who refer to him as "Dr. J."

As a dental expert—licensed in forty-two states as an expert witness—he has been involved in more than one thousand dental malpractice, peer review, and injury cases, making him one of the top-known dental experts in the country. He has published and been written about hundreds of times in print, radio, and on television.

Dr. Grossman is currently a volunteer professor at UCLA School of Dentistry and an adjunct assistant professor at NYU College of Dentistry. Through Homeless Not Toothless, he has made it possible for over 135,000 homeless veterans, victims of domestic abuse, and foster children to receive over $11 million in pro-bono dental care since its inception in 1992 (as of 2023).

He lives with his wife in the Malibu/Thousand Oaks area of Los Angeles, as well as in the Santa Ynez, CA, wine region, has fourteen children, and received a black belt in martial arts at the age of forty-five.

Essential Pillars website for downloads of documents
www.drjaydds.com

Homeless Not Toothless
https://www.homelessnottoothless.org/

Grind Toothpaste
https://grindgoods.com/products/grindtoothpaste

Concierge Dentistry
https://www.conciergedentistry.com/

The *Essential Pillars*—for private coaching, referrals to experts, and to contact the author
www.drjaydds.com

Email for the *Essential Pillars*—for private coaching
EssentialPillars@gmail.com

Additional Reading

I've read countless books and taken thousands of hours of continuing education, all of which has given me a huge advantage in my own success. I have incorporated their ideas into **Essential Pillars**, but I still want to offer, as a resource at least, a partial list of titles I believe may help you as well.

Considering the number of hours it would take to read all of these, I suggest you focus your time on books that tackle your specific weaknesses.

- *Profit First,* by Mike Michalowicz: an excellent deep dive into money management theory.
- *Go for No! Yes Is the Destination, No Is How You Get There,* by Richard Fenton and Andrea Waltz: a brilliant way to handle rejection by getting one yes after going for ten nos!
- *Questions Are the Answer,* by Hal Gregersen: helps you become a person who asks great questions that yield greater answers.
- *Extreme Ownership,* by Jocko Willink and Leif Babin: a decorated Navy SEAL takes the leadership skills he learned in the military over to the business world and shows how to apply them to any team, family, or organization.

- *The E-myth Revisited*, by Michael E. Gerber: about the entrepreneurial mess caused by people who confuse their skills as technicians with their ability to own and run a business.
- *The 7 Habits of Highly Effective People*, by Stephen R. Covey: a deep dive into how habits influence your future and determine whether you will be successful.
- *Atomic Habits*, by James Clear: practical strategies for forming and changing habits. Here's my favorite quote from the book: "People do not decide their futures; they decide their habits, and their habits decide their futures."
- *The One Thing*, by Gary Keller: what is the one thing you must do today that will make a tremendous difference in what you are causing?
- *The 5 Love Languages*, by Gary Chapman: he describes five basic love languages; knowing yours and your significant other's is crucial for success in relationships.
- *Purple Cow*, by Seth Godin: how to make your business stand out and apart from the rest.
- *Never Split the Difference*, by Chris Voss: tools for becoming more persuasive in both your business and personal lives through high-stakes negotiations.
- *Tools of Titans*, by Tim Ferriss: tools and tactics to use in business.
- *Think and Grow Rich*, by Napoleon Hill: the granddaddy of beginner business books, this classic offers thirteen steps toward success.
- *Fix This Next*, by Mike Michalowicz: figuring out your biggest business problem, fixing it, eradicating frustrations, and growing your business.
- *The Ultimate Sales Machine*, by Chet Holmes: how to tune up your business and staff, focusing on "impact areas."

- *Monsters and How to Tame Them,* by Kevin Hart: not the famed comedian's typical stand-up routine, but a guide on how to live your life.
- *Pre-Suasion,* by Robert B. Cialdini: the difference between effective communicators and successful persuaders.
- *The Dip,* by Seth Godin: dives into the low points of business, the setbacks, and the questions to ask.
- *The Talent Code,* by Daniel Coyle: the secret of unlocking talent using "deep practice."
- *Greenlights,* by Matthew McConaughey: the wisdom and lessons learned by the acclaimed actor, and how to live with greater satisfaction.
- *Range,* by David Epstein: performance, success, and education as applied to generalists and specialists.
- *The Price of Tomorrow,* by Jeff Booth: explores the easy access we have to credit and the effects of that on the economy.
- *The Art of Impossible,* by Steven Kotler: secrets of peak performers.
- *The Rise of Superman,* by Steven Kotler: decoding the mystery of ultimate human performance.
- *Lives of the Stoics,* by Ryan Holiday: a look at the people who invented stoic virtues, courage, justice, temperance, and wisdom.
- *Rich Dad Poor Dad,* by Robert T. Kiyosaki: exploring the myth that you need to earn a high income to become rich.
- *Rich Dad's Cashflow Quadrant,* by Robert T. Kiyosaki: an essential read for learning about the four quadrants of earning—employee, small business, big business, and investor.
- *Mating in Captivity,* by Esther Perel: explore the paradoxical union of domesticity and sexual desire.

- *The 80/20 Principle,* by Richard Koch: also known as the Pareto principle, the theory that 80 percent of results come from 20 percent of our efforts.
- *What it Takes,* by Stephen A. Schwarzman: lessons in the pursuit of excellence by the co-founder of Blackstone.
- *Willpower Doesn't Work,* by Benjamin Hardy: nurture is more powerful than nature in creating an environment that does not create and control you.
- *The Miracle Morning,* by Hal Elrod: an essential read! I follow this formula daily—it is a routine designed to get your day set up for you to be powerful.
- *Miracle Morning Millionaires,* by Hal Elrod and David Osborn: practices for creating and transforming your life that begin first thing in the morning.
- *Finite and Infinite Games,* by James P. Carse: distinctions between games that have an end time and those that are infinite, as in the game of life.
- *Shut Up and Listen!,* by Tilman Fertitta: take your company to the next level with coaching from a billionaire restaurant owner who has mastered customer service.
- *Getting to Yes,* by Roger Fisher: four principles for effective negotiation.
- *The 10X Rule,* by Grant Cardone: set targets that are ten times bigger than what you believe you can achieve.
- *See You at the Top,* by Zig Ziglar: getting to the top through honesty, loyalty, faith, integrity, and personal character.
- *How to Make Sh*t Happen,* by Sean Whalen: motivation alone won't do it—this takes work!
- *Can't Hurt Me,* by David Goggins: a decorated soldier in all three branches of the military, the author came from poverty and prejudice and made it big with self-discipline and mental toughness as an ultimate athlete.

- *The Subtle Art of Not Giving a F*ck,* by Mark Manson: a fun read. Personal stories of the author's early traumas point you toward focusing on what really matters.
- *Traction,* by Gino Wickman: a must-read that offers actual methods for solving business problems while explaining why pleasing everyone is a bad idea.
- *Change Your Questions, Change Your Life,* by Marilee Adams: how using the right questions leads to the right answers and wiser solutions.
- *How to Win Friends and Influence People,* by Dale Carnegie: a classic about ways to make people like you, leading to better and healthier relationships and improved business.
- *The Power of Now,* by Eckhart Tolle: how people interact with themselves and others, with exercises for achieving enlightenment.
- *Secrets of the Millionaire Mind,* by T. Harv Eker: dives into the mindset of wealthy people.
- *Pitch Anything,* by Oren Klaff: learn how to pitch your ideas, raise capital, and enroll others in your projects.
- *The Personal MBA,* by Josh Kaufman: an alternative to going to business school.
- *Oversubscribed,* by Daniel Priestley: creating more demand than supply.
- *Money: Master the Game,* by Tony Robbins: the self-help guru interviews legends in the money world and offers a blueprint for securing financial freedom, including setting up a savings and investing plan.
- *The Great Game of Business,* by Jack Stack: sharing financials with employees so they can see what the true costs are can help in controlling overhead and fostering participation in profit-sharing, leading to company growth.

- *Taking Stock,* by Jordan Grumet: originally a hospice doctor, the author gives advice on financial independence and living in the present.
- *Die with Zero,* by Bill Perkins: invest in experiences with the goal of spending down all you have before your final exit.
- *Never Finished,* by David Goggins: explores the power of the mind to blow past "limits."
- *The Magic of Thinking Big,* by David J. Schwartz: similar to Think and Grow Rich, this book discusses how successful people become successful, why others listen to them, and why unsuccessful people use excuses and blame to validate their failures.
- *The Wealthy Gardener,* by John Soforic: the world is a judge that weighs results, not efforts. All dreams are built on the investment of our time.
- *The Psychology of Money,* by Morgan Housel: money has very little to do with intelligence, and everything to do with behavior.

Made in the USA
Coppell, TX
22 January 2025

44772528R00125